Eco-Beau

ECO-BEAUTIFUL

THE ULTIMATE GUIDE TO NATURAL BEAUTY AND WELLNESS

LINA HANSON

PHOTOGRAPHY BY DOVE SHORE

RODALE

© 2009 by Lina Hanson

All rights reserved. No part of this publication may be reproduced or transmitted in any form
or by any means, electronic or mechanical, including photocopying, recording, or any other
information storage and retrieval system, without the written permission of the publisher.

Rodale books may be purchased for business or promotional use or for special sales.
For information, please write to:
Special Markets Department, Rodale Inc., 733 Third Avenue, New York, NY 10017

Printed in the United States of America
Rodale Inc. makes every effort to use acid-free ∞, recycled paper ♲.

Photographs by Dove Shore, with the exception of photographs on pages 61 and 63: © Tyler Boye

Book design by Christina Gaugler

Library of Congress Cataloging-in-Publication Data is on file with the publisher.

ISBN 13: 978–1–60529–881–8

Distributed to the trade by Macmillan

2   4   6   8   10   9   7   5   3   1   paperback

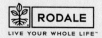

We inspire and enable people to improve their lives and the world around them
For more of our products visit **rodalestore.com** or call 800-848-4735

In memory of my loving grandmother, Lisbeth Hanson,
who taught me that beauty comes from the inside out.

Contents

Acknowledgments   ix

Introduction   xi

Chapter 1: Green Is the New Black   1

Chapter 2: Beauty from the Inside Out   18

Chapter 3: Skin Deep   40

Chapter 4: Eco-Application   64

Chapter 5: The All-Around "Green Guy"   94

Chapter 6: Day and Night Looks   112

Chapter 7: Timeless Eco-Beauty   134

Epilogue   163

Glossary   165

Resources   173

About the Author   179

Index   181

Acknowledgments

I want to thank the following people who helped me along the journey of writing this book. Without your help, this project would not have been possible. You are all eco-beautiful from the inside out!

First and foremost, Steven Priggé, my husband and true friend, who inspired me to write this book and who always makes me feel eco-beautiful. You have enriched my life beyond words. I love you! My tireless agent, Lauren Keller Galit, who understood my vision with this book from the start and helped me make it a reality. We did it! My editor, Julie Will, who continually pushed me to make this book better and better. Thank you for everything! My publicist, Beth Tarson, who went full steam ahead with this book and never looked back. Photographer Dove Shore, whose talent I admire and friendship I cherish. Jeanine Lobell, my mentor and close friend, you not only taught me about makeup, but about life, as well. My agents at Magnet, you are the best! Thank you for your continued support. Mara Roszak and Amy Hollier, the hair goddesses, who make women feel as good as they look. Maelle De

Shutter, the best food stylist around. Food has never looked so good! Lisette Carlsson, my assistant on this book, who helped make things so much smoother and more enjoyable. Raffaele Ruberto of mod.skin labs, whose experience in the field is invaluable. Josie Maran, whose knowledge and approach to being "green" is truly admirable. Fabulous facialist Chanel Jenae, who makes women glow. To all the fabulous models in this book who brightened up the pages with their beauty and spirit.

I would also like to thank my entire family back home in Sweden. You might be far away, but are always in my heart. My best friends and partners in crime, Aki Larsson, Malin Bergman, Genevieve Cortese, Mehera Blum, and Elin Frodin, who always brighten my day. Love you guys! And, last but not least, my dog Madison, who has a knack for making me smile whenever I need it.

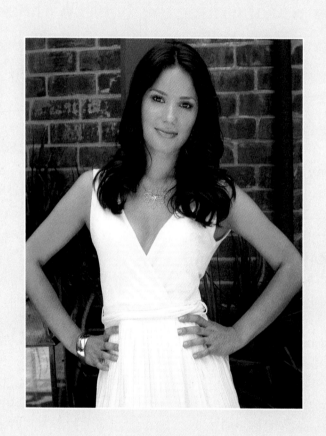

Introduction

I knew from a very young age that I wanted to become a makeup artist. When I was a little girl, I used to sneak into my mother's bathroom and try out all of her new cosmetics. Lipsticks, mascaras, perfumes, blushes, hand creams, body lotions—you name it, I loved it! I was captivated by makeup. I'd spend hours and hours in front of the mirror, copying the techniques and tricks I read about in her glossy fashion magazines.

Eventually I moved to New York City to pursue my passion—a career as a makeup artist. I landed the dream job of assisting makeup artist Jeanine Lobell (the creator of Stila Cosmetics). She took me under her wing and truly taught me the trade. After spending 3 years working alongside Jeanine, I decided to pack my bags, give up my cute apartment in Manhattan, and drive cross-country from New York City to Hollywood. Today, I have a wide-ranging celebrity clientele and I work behind-the-scenes at red-carpet events, fashion shows, magazine shoots, and movie premieres.

Moving from New York City to Los Angeles not only changed my career, it also opened my eyes to a more healthy way of living. Weekend activities like brunching at sidewalk cafés, sipping mocha lattes, and eating fattening quiche were quickly replaced with long hikes up

Runyon Canyon and wholesome lunches of freshly made salads and juices. Trust me, when you go from wearing a bathing suit for 3 months out of the year to 9 months, you get in shape *fast*!

Soon I made even more changes: I began eating organic and locally grown produce, incorporated antioxidants and omega-3 oils into my diet, doubled my daily water intake, and reduced my sugar intake. Not only did my skin improve, but I had increased energy and clarity. And this newfound feeling of well-being made me want to be healthier and more conscious in other aspects of my life.

It also seemed that everywhere I turned, Californians weren't just talking about getting healthy, they were also talking about "going green." How can we help the environment? How can we use less energy? How can we stop global warming? How can each of us start making a difference in our own way? I wondered how *I* could make a difference. It was one thing to green my own life-style—recycle more, drive less, use reusable water bottles—but how could I make my concern for the environment a part of my work, my passion, my every-day trade?

At the same time, I began to notice a distinct shift in the cosmetics industry. Just as nutritionists were discouraging people from eating food that contained a laundry list of unpronounceable ingredients, there was also a heightened awareness of the potentially harmful ingredients found in many cosmetics. I discovered that there are many nasty and toxic ingredients listed right on the packaging of a lot of conventional makeup.

When I switched to an eco-friendly skin-care and makeup regimen, I saw big differences in my own skin almost immediately. I didn't have as many breakouts. The red spots I had had on my cheeks for years disappeared. In fact, my skin was glowing even when I wasn't wearing any makeup at all. That was when I realized how *I* could help the environment every day! Why not start using eco-friendly cosmetics in my practice? And that's exactly what I did.

When I first started doing makeup professionally, I could count on one hand the number of eco-friendly cos-metics products on the market, and they were mostly sold in health food stores—not exactly the sexiest environment for buying makeup. Now there are countless organic, pure mineral, and natural cosmetics companies that offer an impressive array of cosmetics sold everywhere from Sephora to Barneys to Target.

A few years ago, it was tough to get the look you wanted using nothing but "green" cosmetics because so few colors and varieties were available, and not every product worked for everyone. Many women might wonder if they will still be able to get that same look they love when they switch to eco-friendly cosmetics. My answer is, *yes!* You can be eco-friendly and still look beautiful. I call it "eco-beautiful."

Eco-beauty is more than a buzz-word—it's a way of life. Becoming eco-beautiful is about being good to the environment *and* being good to yourself. It's about embracing your inner and outer beauty by using products that are from, quite possibly, the greatest makeup artist of all: Mother Nature. When you nurture your skin with natural products made from ingredients that are actually beneficial to your health, rather than harmful, it will show!

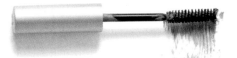

So many people these days pay close attention to what they put in their bodies—but not everyone is as careful about what they put *on* their bodies. I want people to understand that you certainly don't have to sacrifice beauty by going green. There are countless, widely available, high-quality "green" cosmetics products that can help you achieve the look you want. The trick, as with any-thing, is to know how to do it. That's where this book comes in. I will show you some extraordinarily effective techniques for creating any look you desire using only eco-friendly makeup. There's no better feeling in the world than looking your best, feeling your best, and doing your best to help the environment.

Whether I'm creating a red-carpet look for a celebrity attending the Academy Awards, helping a bride look perfect on her wedding day, or glamming up a friend who has a date, it's a new and exciting experience each and every time I pick up a brush. And that's exactly what I want this book to be like for you—a new and exciting experience every time you turn the page.

If there's one important thing I've learned during my years spent working in the makeup industry, it's that to be successful you have to continue to look to the future. And the future is looking more eco-friendly every day. So let's make it eco-beautiful!

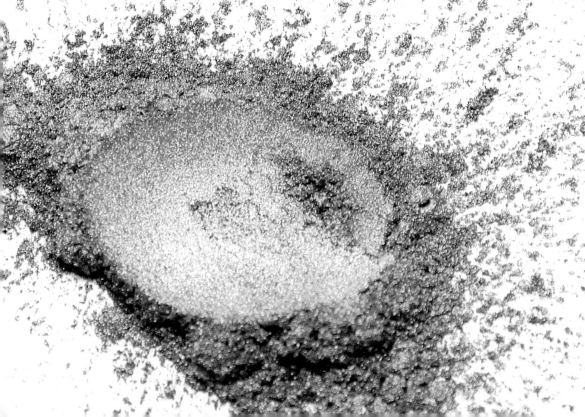

chapter 1

GREEN IS
BLACK

THE NEW

Over the past few years, the "green" movement has hit our world like a tidal wave. From magazines to Web sites to blogs, it's everywhere! Going green requires an active commitment to making the planet a cleaner, better place to live—thereby ensuring a healthy future for everyone.

These days, being green is both fashionable and functional, and for many people—from middle-class moms to movie stars—environmental awareness is an integral part of everyday life. If the 1980s were about excess and the 1990s were about recovering from the 1980s, then the new millennium is about *conservation*.

You've probably heard and seen countless lists of things you can do to help the environment: recycle, decrease your energy usage, eat locally grown produce, shop with reusable canvas bags, own one car (preferably a hybrid), and so on. Hollywood has certainly been at the forefront of this movement. It's next to impossible not to notice celebrities tirelessly advocating worldwide environmental awareness. From Halle Berry opting to use eco-friendly diapers to the cast and crew of *Grey's Anatomy* using thermoses instead of plastic bottles on set, many celebrities are supporting environmental causes.

GETTING GREEN AND GORGEOUS

Some green habits are easier to adopt than others. While taking shorter showers may be a drag, using eco-friendly cosmetics couldn't be more fun! It's a great way to start greening your routine. Products that are made with only natural or botanical ingredients are better for both you *and* the environment. There are so many eco-friendly companies with great products these days. A few of my favorites are Josie Maran Cosmetics, Mod.Skin Labs, Benefit, Dr.Hauschka, and Bare Escentuals, whose slogan is: "Makeup so pure you can sleep in it."

Eco-friendly makeup contains vitamins and powerful antioxidants that will help your skin fight harmful free radicals. What are free radicals? Free radicals are atoms or molecules that contain an extra electron, which causes them to be unstable and to attack cells within the body. The harsh truth is that free radicals are almost every-where—in processed foods, sunlight, cigarette smoke, and quite possibly in the air you're breathing right now. These nasty little suckers can do a number on your skin, causing cellular damage that promotes premature aging. And let's face it, *none* of us are getting any younger. Antioxidants have been proven to help fight the effects of free radicals, and the more, the better! A lot of eco-friendly makeup contains the powerful, free radical–abolishing vitamins A, C, and E. So not only will you look sexy on the outside, you'll also absorb these essential vitamins into your body. With eco-friendly makeup you get healthier with every stroke of the brush!

Eco-friendly makeup is good for every skin type, but it's particularly good for "problem" skin. I always tell women that one of the best things about using eco-friendly cosmetics is that it puts them in control of their own skin.

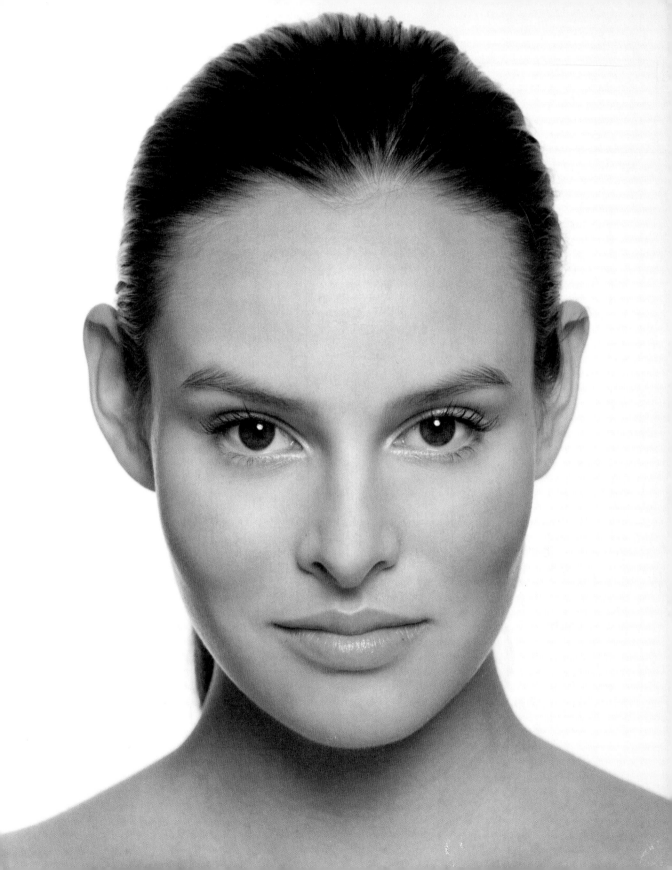

For example, I have a friend in her thirties who has suffered for years with rosacea, which can create symptoms like puffiness and redness of the cheeks, chin, nose, and forehead. Her case was mild, but still noticeable enough to make her feel self-conscious. I suggested that she start incorporating mineral makeup into her daily beauty regimen. The anti-inflammatory properties in mineral makeup made a big difference. In just a little over a month, the redness caused by her rosacea decreased tremendously. The makeup allowed her skin to breathe rather than be suffocated with heavy, caked-on foundation to hide the problem. She found a new makeup regimen that she loves and, more importantly, she developed a newfound confidence in herself.

Eco-friendly makeup comes in so many varieties that it can be hard to know which formula or product is right for you. Here's what you need to know to make the right purchases.

Mineral Makeup

There has been so much talk about mineral makeup over the last few years—it's taking the beauty world by storm. Mineral makeup is made up of hypoallergenic loose powders that naturally nourish and enhance the skin with 100 percent pure minerals like titanium, gold, zinc, magnesium, and aluminum. These products contain none of the perfumes, dyes, talc, alcohol, mineral oil, or preservatives that can be found in most conventional makeup formulas.

The great thing about mineral makeup is that it truly works for all skin types. It's *especially* good for women with

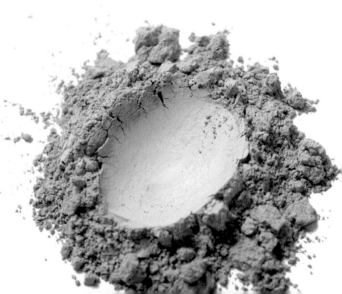

ultra-sensitive skin. Women who suffer from acne, dryness, clogged pores, or other skin problems find that mineral makeup actually enhances their skin tone rather than exacerbating existing problems or creating new ones. Mineral makeup never feels like a mask on your skin. The small, lightweight pigments in the minerals bind the skin together—the result is a beautiful complexion with a radiant, natural glow.

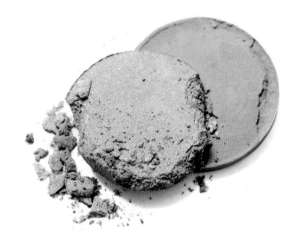

Why is mineral makeup so good for you? Simply put, the ingredients in mineral makeup come from the earth, not from a factory. Does it work as effectively as conventional cosmetics do? In my experience, mineral powder foundations actually offer the same great coverage as traditional liquid foundation. What I love best about mineral makeup is that it's so light and clean on the skin, you can mix and match it, and it never looks too heavy. It's so much fun! That said, be conservative and take your time when you first try it. Applying mineral makeup prop-erly takes some getting used to. But don't worry—I'll share all of my favor-ite techniques with you in Chapter 4!

Organic and Certified Organic Makeup

Like mineral makeup, organic cosmet-ics are becoming more and more popular. And because they also contain ingredients that are natural and non-drying, they work for all skin types. The ingredients used in organic makeup either come directly from plants or are substances derived from plant materi-als. The term *organic* refers to the agricultural practices used to grow and process the ingredients in a product. All of the active ingredients in organic makeup are grown without chemicals or pesticides.

Just because a product is labeled "organic" or "natural" doesn't necessarily mean it's certified organic, however. When in doubt, look for the trusty USDA Organic logo. According to industry regulations, if the packaging claims that the product is organic, it must contain at least 95 percent organic ingredients. If it says "made with organic ingredients," then at least 70 percent or more of the product was made with organic ingredients, though the inactive ingredients may not be organic. Any cosmetic product labeled "Certified Organic" contains 100 percent organic ingredients. Absolutely no synthetic chemicals may be used at any stage of the production chain, from the growing to the harvesting, storage, transporting, and processing stages. The ingredients must be naturally extracted plant products and may not be genetically modified.

Organic makeup isn't difficult to find. There are many fabulous companies that offer a wide array of products. Two of my favorites are Josie Maran Cosmetics and Jane Iredale. Certified organic makeup can be a bit tougher to find and is not always available in makeup stores. You can order online from great brands like Miessence and the Organic Make-up Company, which carry full selections of products from foundations to lip glosses and everything in between.

Natural Makeup

Natural makeup is made without the addition of synthetic additives like chemical preservatives, colors, or fragrances. The majority of the ingredients in natural makeup are derived from plant extracts and/or natural ingredients. However, unlike organic makeup, the ingredients may be grown with pesticides and are *not* certified organic.

Keep in mind that there is no official definition of the term "natural" as it applies to cosmetics. Some products that are labeled "natural" could still use synthetics for preservation. Remember to check the label thoroughly. You have to take the manufacturer's word for it that the ingredients are natural. I recommend MyChelle and Physicians Formula products.

There are plenty of natural makeup companies that offer a complete line for a full-face makeover—foundations, bronzers, eye shadow, mascara, blushes, lipsticks, lip pencils, and lip glosses. It doesn't matter what skin type or skin tone you have, the foundations, shadows, and lipsticks all come in a wide range of colors and shades to get you looking better than ever.

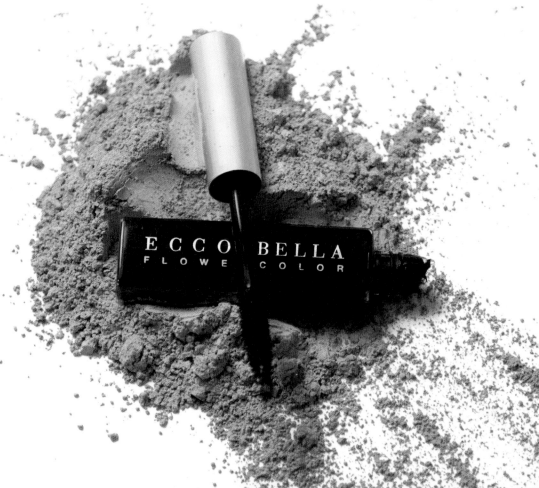

A CONSCIOUS COSMETICS LINE

Josie Maran is one of the most famous models in the world, but she grew up far from the spotlight, living a bohemian childhood in northern California. Her mother never wore makeup, which inspired Josie to take a natural approach to beauty herself. Josie began her modeling career at age 12 and found huge success. She landed on the cover of *Glamour* magazine six times, had a stint as the iconic Guess girl, and was featured in the *Sports Illustrated* swimsuit issue 3 years in a row. While working in the fashion industry, Josie began to look at cosmetics a bit differently. "As I began to land jobs, I discovered what a lot of other girls already knew: the power of makeup," reflects Josie. "I was surprised to see how makeup could transform not just my look but also my mood!"

In 1997, Josie became the face of Maybelline, a title she held for nearly a decade. However, becoming a mother inspired Josie to launch her own eco-friendly makeup company, Josie Maran Cosmetics (josiemarancosmetics.com). It is truly a chic and "conscious" cosmetics line, made of eco-friendly ingredients and housed in biodegradable packaging. I talked with Josie about her makeup line and the importance of using eco-friendly cosmetics.

How were you first introduced to a "green" lifestyle?

I was born into a family that cares about environmental and social issues, so you could say my awareness of environmental issues was just a natural part of my upbringing. Having a daughter of my own has led me to a whole new "eco-awakening"—inspiring me to be even more conscious of our impact on the environment.

Why was creating an eco-friendly makeup line so important to you?

I was pregnant around the same time I was developing the line, and it definitely made me more aware of what I was putting inside my body and on my skin. It made me even more adamant about not using any products that contain parabens or petrochemicals or fragrances.

In your opinion, what are the major benefits of eco-friendly cosmetics?

The major benefit is knowing that while you are enhancing your beauty you are not harming your health. Putting unhealthy chemicals on your skin day in, day out, is really creating a major health problem.

These days, do you think women are becoming more environmentally friendly and aware of eco-friendly beauty?

There is so much info now about the planet and how we need to change the way we think and act. I think women are becoming very aware of how much of an impact they have and I do see many women making eco-friendly changes.

Why should women use eco-friendly cosmetics?

There are wonderful, safe, and nourishing ingredients in eco-friendly makeup.

The company which creates the eco-friendly makeup is coming from a conscious place. You do not have to sacrifice great makeup for your health anymore!

Oh So Good Oil

Every woman should keep **Josie Maran Cosmetics' Argan Oil** on hand at all times. Organically grown in Morocco, this lightweight oil is rich in vitamin E and fatty acids and can be used for a variety of beauty needs, from split ends to dry cuticles. And it comes in a recyclable glass bottle. You've just struck oil, ladies!

BE ON THE LOOKOUT

Even if you're looking in the right makeup categories, read *all* of the ingredients listed on the package. The Chemical Safe Skincare Campaign reports that the average woman uses 12 toiletries every day and applies more than 175 chemical compounds to her body in the process. Many of these chemicals have been known to cause various skin problems. Furthermore, Chemical Safe states that 60 percent of skin-care ingredients end up being absorbed into the body. The group is demanding that cosmetics companies improve the information on their product labels.

I recently got a voice-mail message from my friend Malin who was excited to tell me about a two-for-one lipstick sale going on at a local drugstore. She said she had bought eight lipsticks in various colors. Yikes! I called Malin back and asked if she had read the ingredients label. She hadn't. Now,

Malin is a personal trainer and I know she watches what she eats religiously. So I explained it to her in a way I knew she'd understand: "You read food labels at the supermarket, right? Well, the same goes for conventional cosmetics." She said she'd never heard of any of the ingredients listed on the packaging—so I asked her if she had kept the receipt. When she said yes, I said, "Return them, girlfriend!"

In September 2007, the Campaign for Safe Cosmetics conducted a study of lead content in lipstick. The shocking findings were that 20 of the 33 brand-name lipsticks tested contained detectable levels of lead. Are you ready for something even scarier? None of these lipsticks listed lead as an ingredient. According to the federal Agency for Toxic Substances and Disease Registry (ATSDR), exposure to high levels of lead can cause pregnant women to have miscarriages. These days, most pregnant women I know use only natural makeup because they know that what they put on their bodies is absorbed through the skin and can affect their babies, too.

Some products will make their health claims loud and clear—but the ones that are bad for you aren't exactly posting their dangers in 20-point type. There are many toxic ingredients to lookout for when reading the packages of conventional makeup. Here are a few you should always avoid.

*Propylene glycol. Used in moisturizers, it's derived from petroleum oil, which is found in automatic brakes and industrial defrosters. Propylene glycol is toxic and may damage cell membranes, causing redness, rashes, and dry skin. Even worse, it can penetrate your skin and enter your bloodstream.

*Sodium lauryl sulphate (SLS). It's used as a thickener and foaming agent in shampoos, toothpastes, and cleansers, and also as a wetting agent in garage floor cleaners, engine and auto degreasers, and auto cleaning products.

SLS can dissolve the oils on your skin, which can cause the skin to separate and create fine lines and wrinkles.

*Coal tar dyes. These can be found in lipstick and have produced cancer in laboratory animals.

*Parabens. These are used to prolong the shelf life of makeup and exhibit strong estrogenic activity in laboratory studies and have been shown to be transdermal (easily absorbed into the bloodstream through the skin). Parabens have also been found in many samples of breast cancer tissue.

Look for the words "paraben free" on any cosmetic label. While there is no conclusive evidence that parabens cause cancer and the cosmetics industry insists that parabens are safe, why take a chance? If there is a safe alternative available with no negative cloud surrounding it, then that's where my product loyalties will lie. I urge you to look not just at the front label, but at the back as well. That's where the *real* story is told.

GOOD THINGS COME IN SMART PACKAGES

I don't know about you, but I'm a sucker for cute cosmetics packaging. I remember when Stila first came on the market. Their adorable drawings of those cute Stila girls really caught my eye, but more importantly, I noticed that the boxes were made of recyclable paper. As it turns out, most of Stila's packaging is made from recycled paper, aluminum, and glass. In fact, they were one of the first mainstream cosmetics companies to house their products in environmentally safe packages. Talk about a trendsetter!

When it comes to buying eco-friendly cosmetics, packaging should be taken into consideration. More and more cosmetics companies are beginning to use packaging that is biodegradable and/or recyclable. They are even striving to make their display units eco-friendly!

My favorite example of this innovation is a product called PlantLove botanical lipstick made by cosmetics company Cargo. The entire package is environmentally friendly—the product contains no mineral oils or petroleum, the recycled paper box is embedded with real flower seeds, and the biodegradable tube is made out of *corn*! I gave my friend Elin a PlantLove lipstick for her birthday. Not only did she love the lipstick, but when she moistened the packaging, planted it in a pot, and put it on her windowsill, she grew beautiful flowers.

Love Me Two Times

Two dollars from the sale of every PlantLove lipstick is donated to Cargo's charity of choice, St. Jude Children's Research Hospital. Great lipstick and a great cause!

BRUSH WITH GREATNESS

Your new eco-beautiful routine should include brushes that are "cruelty free," meaning they are not made from animal hair. Always opt for brushes made of synthetic hair. These brushes are durable as well as extremely soft and luxurious. And you can get all the brushes you need in this eco-friendly format—powder brush, fan brush, eye shadow brush, blush brush, lip brush—you name it! Walgreens sells a top-notch, affordable collection of brushes called EcoTools (parispresents.com). It doesn't get better than that—budget friendly, eco-friendly, and easy to find. Additionally, Hourglass Cosmetics (hourglasscosmetics.com) offers PETA-friendly bristles on their line of brushes.

In fact, the Hourglass blush brush made it onto *Elle* magazine's 2008 Green Stars product list.

Don't underestimate the power of your brushes. A friend of mine complained about clogged pores. She would often get breakouts, especially on her chin. I put her on a completely organic makeup regimen. Her skin certainly got better, but she still suffered from clogged pores. Hmmm. I began to think hard about what could be causing her skin problems. Because she always came to my place to get her makeup done, one day I suggested going to her house. As soon as I walked into her bathroom I found the culprit behind her clogged pores and breakouts—dirty makeup brushes!

The Brush-Off

The more frequently you clean your brushes, the longer they will last. I suggest doing brush maintenance once every 2 weeks. If you're a party girl, do it once a week!

Dirty makeup brushes are a breeding ground for bacteria. In between the bristles of a brush, dirt, facial oils, and old makeup can really accumulate. I immediately showed her the best way to do brush maintenance. In my opinion, regular brush cleaners are much too harsh and the residue they leave behind could make you break out even more. Here is my gentle, natural method for keeping makeup brushes clean.

1. Run the bristles of the brush under lukewarm water.

2. Apply a small amount of eco-friendly dishwashing liquid (such as Seventh Generation or Method) to the bristles and work into a lather. These cleaning solutions are nontoxic, hypoallergenic, and not tested on animals.

3. Rinse the brush thoroughly under the water for a couple of minutes, until all of the bristles have returned to their natural color.

4. Lay the brush on a clean, dry towel and let it air dry.

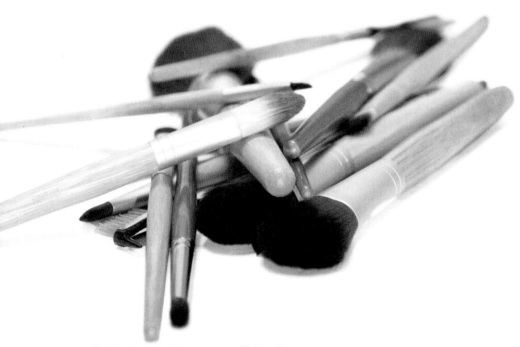

A CHANGE WILL DO YOU GOOD

Sheryl Crow sang it and I really believe it holds true. A change can do all of us good when it comes to creating a new look. However, for most women, taking that first step outside of their comfort zone seems to be the most difficult part.

Humans are creatures of habit, especially when it comes to our appearance. We are often afraid to try something new, be creative, or mix it up. Have you been applying your makeup the same way for the past decade? Have you been wearing the same perfume since the Reagan administration? Are you creating the same makeup look day after day out of habit, afraid to try something new? If so, I have news for you—you're in a makeup rut. I have many clients, as well as friends and family members, who have fallen victim to a makeup rut. It's quite easy to do. You have a makeup drawer filled with foundations, blushes, glosses, and shadows that you know will do the job. You

buy your products at the same store and keep using the same ones over and over again. You have your day look and your evening look down pat. Well, I have one word for you . . . BORING!

Makeup is supposed to be fresh and exciting. Trying eco-friendly makeup gives you the perfect opportunity to get out of that rut and experiment with something different while doing something good for your body. In fact, many of the companies that make your favorite tried-and-true products are going eco-friendly. L'Oréal, one of the cosmetics industry's oldest and most trusted companies, has announced recently that it's coming out with a mineral makeup line.

I recommend easing into a new routine. Go to a store you like, such as Sephora, Macy's, Nordstrom, or another department store, and experiment with a new eco-friendly lipstick shade or a new mineral blush. Find a product line that works for you by trying out one or two new products. If you like what you see—which I'm sure you will—then slowly begin incorporating eco-friendly makeup from the rest of that line into your beauty routine.

I've written this book to help you make that transition, so keep reading, and keep an open mind. Don't be afraid to play with your makeup.

You'll be surprised to see what a new eco-friendly eye pencil or eye shadow can do for you. No matter what season it is, start with a spring cleaning of your makeup bag to make room for the new products that you'll fit into your new routine. Still not convinced? Here is a recap of my top eight reasons why you should get eco-beautiful.

EIGHT IS ENOUGH

1. **Healthy from the outside in**. If you worry about what you put in your body, then you should worry about what you put *on* your body.

2. **You get what you pay for**. It's an old adage, but it still holds true. Eco-friendly makeup costs a bit more than some conventional varieties, but it's chock-full of vitamins and enzymes that are essential if you want your skin to get that gorgeous glow. Your extra investment will produce big results.

3. **Anti-aging**. Aging is one thing that we are *all* unanimously "anti." Eco-friendly makeup has many anti-aging properties to help fight against the effects of free radicals and other causes of premature aging.

4. **Look good and do good**. Eco-friendly makeup works just as well as your favorite old brands—and there's nothing like looking good and doing something good for the environment at the same time.

5. **Better on than off**. Eco-friendly makeup is filled with so many vitamins that it's actually better for your skin than not wearing makeup at all.

6. **Oh, baby.** Pregnant women are choosing natural makeup because they know that what they put on their bodies is absorbed through their skin and can affect their babies.

7. **Cruelty free**. If you are an animal lover like me, you will be happy to know that eco-friendly cosmetics companies only sell products that have not been tested on animals.

8. **Commitment.** Eco-friendly companies have made a commitment to health. They are going beyond the marketing gimmicks. For them, the proof is in the product.

chapter 2

BEAUTY
FROM THE
INSIDE OUT

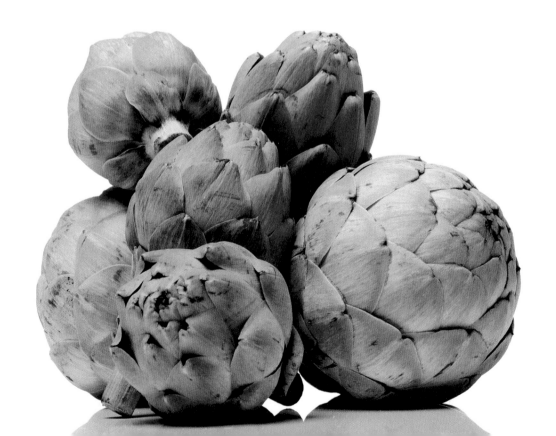

Growing up in Sweden certainly taught me how to live the healthy lifestyle I choose today. I grew up in a small town 3 hours north of Stockholm. From a young age, I learned about the importance of eating fresh, nutritious foods. My family ate locally grown produce and a lot of fresh fish. We lived on one of the three biggest lakes in Sweden and my dad and I used to go fishing in the summer and bring our catches home for dinner. We'd pick mushrooms and berries and make soups, stews, and jams. Sugar and soda were no-no's in our house. And because I never had them—I never missed them!

This healthy lifestyle during my childhood helped me stay conscious of what I ate when I moved to the United States. I immediately noticed that the portions in American restaurants were far bigger than what I was accustomed to back home. I was also surprised to see 50 different types of sugary cereal in the grocery store. Doughnut shops, fast-food chains, ice cream parlors—sugar seemed to be everywhere. These days, luckily, people have become much more health conscious. Terms such as *antioxidant* are now buzzwords in the marketing of food and beauty products. I am happy to say that this *isn't* just a gimmick. Antioxidants are vital to the prevention of cellular damage, which is a common cause of disease and aging.

I believe different dietary lifestyles work for different people. It's important to find things you like that work for your body type. I know that whichever dietary road you choose, it is important to find the right antioxidant-rich foods within that diet. What we put in our bodies has an enormous effect on how we feel and how our skin looks. I can show you all the makeup tips and tricks in the world, but wholesome, nutritious foods are the true foundation for beautiful skin.

ANTI-AGING EATS

It has been said that in this world nothing is certain, except death and taxes. I think they should add wrinkles to that list. While they may be inevitable, there are things you can do to lessen the appearance of fine lines and wrinkles.

You've probably heard this before, but the body *is* just like a car—you have to put in the right fuel in order for it to run smoothly and efficiently. You can use all the fancy miracle wrinkle creams in the world, but there is no substitute for healthy food to keep your skin looking youthful. A diet rich in antioxidants is key to fighting off the free radicals that can cause premature aging.

Boiling Point

In a study conducted by the American Botanical Council, 80 percent of the raw antioxidant power in vegetables was maintained when they were steamed, but only 30 percent was maintained after boiling.

Contrary to popular belief, a woman can't live on frozen yogurt and sushi alone. A diet packed with power foods high in calcium, magnesium, iron, zinc, vitamin C, vitamin E, and beta-carotene can drastically reduce aging, keep your hair shiny, prevent disease, and bring overall wellness and energy to the mind and body.

The following antioxidant-rich foods will feed your skin from the inside out. Put these on your next grocery list and, as always, try to buy organic.

Best Beauty Foods

Artichokes. These are extremely high in vitamin C, which helps provide proper blood circulation—one of the best ways to fight skin aging. Researchers at the USDA ranked artichokes as the top antioxidant vegetable, surpassing spinach and broccoli.

Beans. Beans are an amazing source of protein and are low in calories. They're also chock-full of antioxidants and hyaluronic acid—an acid that

naturally occurs in the skin and helps to retain moisture. A lack of hyaluronic acid in the body is known to spark premature aging. Eat beans three to four times a week and your levels will be covered.

Beetroot. This prime purple food contains anthocyanins, which are antioxidant flavonoids that help promote collagen production in the body. Eating beetroot is like an all-natural collagen injection. Look out, Dr. 90210!

Blueberries. Blueberries have the best power food combination: They're low in sugar and high in antioxidants. They also have anti-inflammatory properties, so wrinkles beware! I love

Oatmeal makes a great breakfast, and it's a quality source of iron and fiber for women. It will also help maintain blood-sugar levels and curb your appetite so you don't reach for unhealthy snacks later in the day.

blueberries in smoothies, on cereal, or just as a snack by themselves.

Brown rice. We all need some carbohydrates to survive, but it's important to eat the *right* carbs. Brown rice is high in B vitamins. So it's great if you're stressed—and we all know how stress can affect our skin. Replace your favorite white flour products with brown rice, and you

won't feel like you need a nap at the end of your next meal.

Cranberries. Like blueberries, cranberries have anti-inflammatory properties. Another reason they made my list is because it's helpful for women to drink unsweetened cranberry juice during their menstrual cycles, as it cleans out the urinary tract and helps prevent infection.

Goji berries. Vitamin C helps the body produce collagen in the skin, and these little berries are packed with 500 times more vitamin C per ounce than oranges are. Goji berries are also high in linoleic acid, which is an essential fat that plumps up the skin and keeps it looking young. Eat them

Snack Attack

When it's midday and you're feeling lethargic and you catch yourself reaching for a sugary snack, try some trail mix instead. I adore Bliss Mix by Transition Nutrition (royalhimalayan.com). It is an amazing raw organic mix of pistachios, Himalayan raisins, mulberries, goji berries, cashews, and more. Keep this in your purse for a natural boost!

by themselves or toss them in a salad. *Yum*.

Kale. This dark green vegetable ignites the liver to produce enzymes that detoxify the body. This is sure to help make your skin and eyes clear. Kale is widely praised as one of the most powerful foods to fight off toxins in the body.

Prunes. High in fiber and antioxidants, prunes give wrinkles a run for their money. In fact, prunes got the highest antioxidant score from USDA scientists at Tufts University, beating out blueberries, blackberries, and apples. Prunes aren't just for grandparents any longer.

Sweet potatoes. This delicious vegetable gets good marks from nutritionists because it's high in nutrients and low in calories. Sweet potatoes contain a large serving of vitamin A, which is a major force in the renewal of skin cells and a key component in the fight against wrinkles. Sweet potatoes also contain a solid amount of calcium, vitamin C, and potassium.

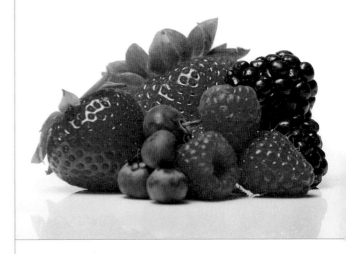

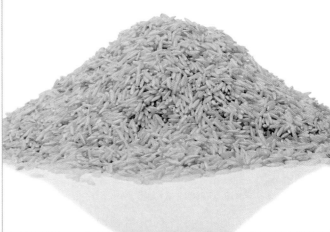

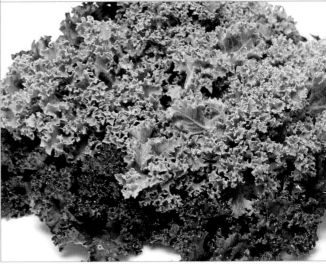

ESSENTIAL OILS

Greece has always been a big resort destination for Swedes. It's a short 3-hour flight, and I vacationed there with my girlfriends during the summer months. I always marveled at how amazing Greek women's skin looked. They weren't afraid to spend time in the strong Mediterranean sun, yet their faces didn't appear to be over-exposed or sun damaged. They all had something that my friends and I called the "Greek glow." In countries like Greece and Italy, where they incorporate a lot of olive oil into their diets, it's clearly doing wonders for the elasticity of their skin.

Oils lubricate the skin from the inside out. When you consume such essential oils as olive, fish, coconut and flaxseed, you are on your way to achieving that same beautiful glow. These oils really help in the fight against wrinkles. Skin cells have a special fatty layer made of omega-3 acids. The more omega-3 acids you have in your body, the stronger the layer of fat will be around the skin cells. The result? Your skin will be plumper and the appearance of wrinkles and lines will be reduced.

Olive, fish, and flaxseed oils, all of which are high in omega-3 acids, can be put on salads, ingested alone, and applied externally. Remember, moderation is key—even good fats can become bad in excess. But if you take them a few times a week, you will see an overall difference.

Twice Is Nice

Twice a week, put a few drops of 14,000 IU pure vitamin E oil in your hands, rub it around, and apply it to your face and neck. This will keep your skin smooth, soft, and hydrated, as well as help prevent discoloration and sun damage.

Organic extra-virgin olive oil. This will help with dry skin from the inside out. Use as a salad dressing with a touch of fresh lemon juice and it will be delish. Besides the internal benefits, olive oil is great to use topically on your skin, hair, and even your nails.

Flaxseed oil. It's a major vegetable source of omega-3 fatty acids. Many medical doctors prescribe flaxseed oil for dry skin, and many dermatologists recommend using it for acne and scars. Organic ground flaxseed meal is another great way to add fiber, fatty acids, and lignans to your skin. Put it on cereals or in smoothies.

Omega-3 fish oil. This fish oil is a dietary source of essential fatty acids that help in the fight against wrinkles. Omega-3s also help burn fat while giving your skin a healthy glow. I suggest taking Nordic Naturals Ultimate Omega fish oil soft gels (nordicnaturals.com).

Coconut oil. I highly suggest using virgin (unprocessed) coconut oil when

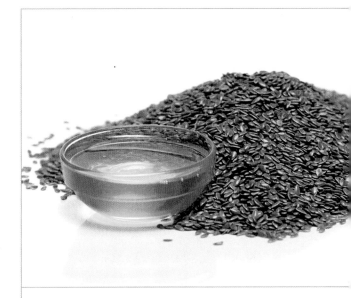

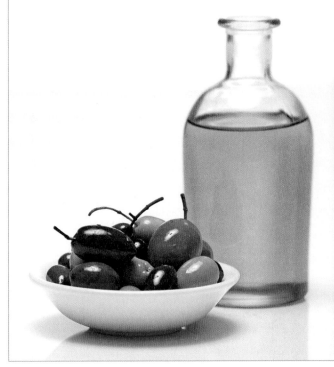

cooking. Unlike some other oils, it doesn't develop trans fat when it is heated. Keep in mind that you buy coconut oil as a solid and it turns into a liquid when it hits approximately 75°F. You can find coconut oil at your local health food store or online (royalhimalayan.com).

COFFEE TALK

There has been an ongoing debate about whether coffee is good or bad for your health. To sip or not to sip—that is the question! Some researchers say coffee is high in antioxidants. Others say coffee drains the body of minerals like calcium. We all know that coffee contains caffeine, and that caffeine is a stimulant. Coffee probably helped you pull an all-nighter back in college to get that term paper done, but I'm afraid when it comes to beauty, caffeine is *not* part of the equation.

Caffeine is a diuretic, meaning that it elevates your rate of urination. This constant expelling of fluids can cause dehydration in the body—and dehydrated skin will undoubtedly lead to fine lines and wrinkles. Also, caffeine wears on your adrenal glands because of the constant stimulation. If your adrenal glands are worn out, you'll feel exhausted and look exhausted. Your skin will appear pale and tired instead of glowing and gorgeous. Also, be wary of the new trend of putting caffeine in beauty products. Various companies are using caffeine in eye creams and claim-ing that it helps to reduce puffiness. While it may decrease puffiness, it also dries out your delicate under-eye skin, which is the most sensitive skin on your entire body!

Caffeine is also known to create a variety of negative physical and mental side effects, such as heartburn, high blood pressure, irritability, anxiety, halitosis (bad breath), and tooth stain-ing. Yellow teeth are *not* eco-beautiful!

Right now you may be saying to yourself, "Okay, then I'll just drink decaffeinated coffee." Unfortunately, that's also a bad idea. Decaffeinated coffee can increase stomach acid as well as specific levels of cholesterol in the blood that can have a harmful effect on the heart. Some people also get head-aches from decaf.

When I lowered my coffee intake, not only did my sleep patterns improve, but my complexion did as well. Not to

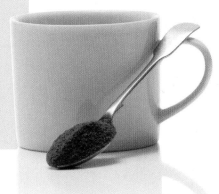

mention all of the money I saved by ending my $4-a-day Starbucks addiction. Let's take a moment to do the math: $4 a day ✕ 365 days a year = $1,460. That's an island getaway with the girls! When I stopped drinking coffee the biggest thing I missed was the actual taste. I adore a hot organic tea, but on those mornings when I have to be on set at 6 a.m., it's just not the same thing. For months I was on the lookout for something that could satisfy my coffee craving. One day, while working on a photo shoot, the photographer recommended that I try something called Dandy Blend. I was skeptical, but after a few sips I found my new morning must-have.

Dandy Blend (dandyblend.com) is chock-full of flavor, courtesy of some simple yet antioxidant-rich ingredients: roasted barley, rye, chicory root, beetroot, and dandelion root. It's also gluten free, sugar free, caffeine free, fat free, and pesticide free, but definitely *not* taste free. Dandy Blend has that dark, smoky, sweet flavor I missed from my morning cup of joe. And the sweet taste doesn't come from any artificial ingredients or sweeteners, but from the fructose that occurs naturally in roasted dandelion and chicory roots. There's also no acidity or bitterness, so no more upset stomach. Give it a try and it'll become your must-have morning beverage in no time!

Puff Daddy

Have you noticed that your eyes and face are sometimes puffy the morning after a big dinner? That's because your body retains water when you eat a lot of salt. Flush out your system and reduce puffiness by drinking lots of water. And at home, you might think about replacing your table salt with organic kelp granules. They come in a handy shaker and add a salty flavor to food without adding a lot of sodium to your diet—or puffiness to your face. They're a great alternative if you have high blood pressure, as well.

WATER WORKS

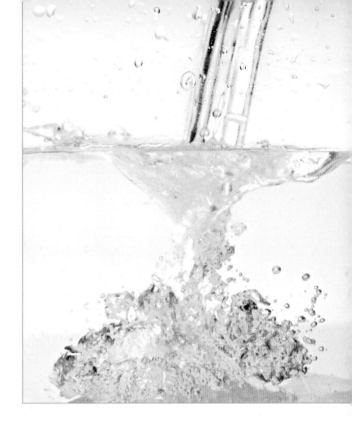

Water is the nectar of the beauty gods. Since the beginning of time, drinking plenty of water has always been a key to having clear and radiant skin. The philosophy behind it is quite simple— water detoxifies the skin by flushing out and getting rid of unwanted waste and harmful toxins in the body. Toxins build up in the body over time, and if they aren't removed from the body, they can secrete through the pores in your skin.

Do you suffer from acne? Are you drinking enough water? You see where I am going here. There is a direct correlation between breakouts and not drinking enough water. If you suffer from acne you should stay far away from fried foods, saturated fats, and alcohol—and drink lots of water! Water also helps prevent the skin from sagging. Mind you, drinking water is not going to cure all of your skin problems, but it's certainly an essential building block on the journey to clear and healthy looking skin. And it's

all about consistency. You should aim to drink the same amount of water every day. How much water should you drink per day? My rule of thumb is one quart for every 50 pounds of body weight.

On a physical level, if you often feel dizzy or fatigued, or if you have been getting headaches on a frequent basis, you probably are not consuming enough water. Water will increase your energy level and improve mental clarity, as well. For a different way to drink your daily water, I suggest trying hot water with organic lemon slices. It's fabulous for digestion and it will aid in the detoxification process.

As of late, there has been much discussion about drinking water out of glass versus plastic bottles. It has been widely reported that using the same plastic bottle over and over again could make you ill, not to mention all of the unnecessary environmental waste. Glass can be washed and reused and can be recycled much more easily than plastic. If you drink out of a glass bottle, you will also really taste the difference.

If you find it difficult to carry around a glass bottle, you should try drinking out of a thermos. I recommend picking up a SIGG (mysigg.com) eco-friendly reusable water bottle. They are 100 percent recyclable, come in lots of fun designs, and only cost a little over $20. Also, SIGG is a member of the organization 1% For The Planet, giving 1 percent of all of its sales to environmental causes.

TROPICAL DELIGHT

Speaking of water, I want to tell you about one of my all-time faves—coconut water. Found in fresh green coconuts, it is extremely high in vital minerals, natural sodium, and potassium. In fact, it has more potassium than a banana.

Coconut water has many vital health benefits: It promotes weight loss, boosts your immune system, and helps digestion. Even though it tastes sweet, coconut water is actually quite low in sugar and calories (16.7 calories per 3.5 ounces).

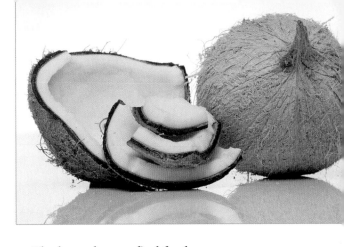

What are its beauty benefits? I've found that drinking coconut water on a regular basis makes my nails stronger and my hair incredibly shiny. It even works on blemishes. Just dab some fresh coconut water directly on a pimple and it will reduce the inflammation and help to prevent scarring. Also, because it's rich in plant protein and replenishes minerals and electrolytes needed by the body, it's a post-workout dream. My advice is to stop drinking those sugary sports drinks that can cause breakouts and go for pure coconut water. It's nature's very own energy drink!

The best place to find fresh green coconuts is your local health food store or natural foods market. However, if you can't locate them there, the next best thing is to try a drink called O.N.E. (onecoco.com). O.N.E. is 100 percent all-natural coconut water packed in individual 11-ounce environmentally friendly Tetra Paks. This drink is easy for you to carry. No excuses—drink up!

NOT SO SWEET

We all like the taste of sugar, but it's not so sweet for your mind and body. A diet high in sugar can affect your sleep as well as your mood. And it's not good for your skin. Sugar is an inflammatory and it damages collagen in your body, which can cause fine lines and wrinkles.

Furthermore, the surge of insulin that sugar causes in your bloodstream can cause breakouts. I urge my clients to read food labels regularly. It might say "sugar free" on the package, but that doesn't mean there isn't a different form of sweetener inside. Look out for ingredients like corn syrup, barley malt, molasses, and artificial flavors, among others.

Many people avoid sugar to lose weight and they use artificial sweeteners as an alternative. There have been conflicting reports about whether or not artificial sweeteners cause health problems, but my advice is to stay away from them altogether. Luckily, there are some great all-natural sweeteners you can use in place of sugar. You can still have your cake and eat it, too! Here are a few of my favorites.

Agave nectar. This all-natural sweetener comes from the agave plant. It won't cause the spike or drop in blood-glucose levels that cane sugar does. Agave can also boost your immune system.

Stevia. This nontoxic sweetener can be found in liquid or powder form. It contains beneficial ingredients such as vitamin C, calcium, beta-carotene, fiber, and potassium, and it actually sweetens *without* calories.

Honey. It's great for digestion and

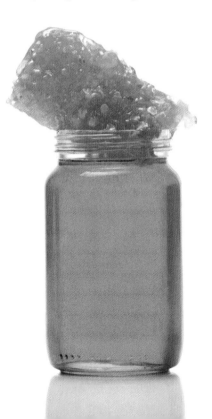

good for your heart. Make sure you use a high-quality honey, and always look for local varieties, which will taste fresh and flavorful.

Organic maple syrup. This is very high in zinc and magnesium, both of which boost your immune system. It also contains vitamins B_2, B_5, and B_6.

Another fabulous replacement for sugar is cinnamon. This rich spice will give your meal added sweetness with none of the breakouts, fine lines, or wrinkles. In fact, cinnamon is one of the spices with the *most* anti-aging

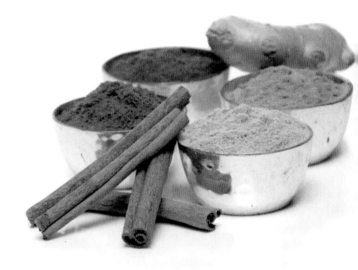

properties. It's tasty and it turns back the clock. Now, that's what I call a win–win situation! For more information on cinnamon, turn to page 34.

SPICE GIRL

One way to spice up your diet and help your skin look its best is to add herbs and spices. Scientific studies suggest that organically grown spices such as oregano, rosemary, turmeric, and cayenne can actually slow down the aging process.

Cooking meals with salt and butter certainly won't get you that eco-beauti-ful glow. Those ingredients may add flavor to your meal, but they also add sodium and saturated fat. Instead, try cooking with organic spices. The meal you love can taste just as delicious—or even better—if you swap salt, fats, and oils for fresh herbs and spices. Here is a list of some antioxidant-rich, anti-aging spices that I strongly suggest using on a

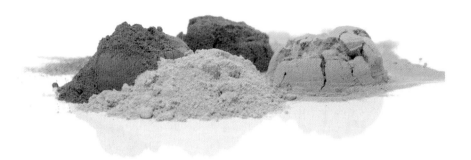

daily basis. Make sure these spices are *always* on your spice rack, because a dash here and a sprinkle there can really go a long way!

- **Turmeric.** A major anti-inflammatory that has been said to act as a sunscreen for the skin from the inside out. Also, it's great for back pain.

- **Oregano.** This super spice has over 40 times the antioxidant power of apples.

- **Ginger.** Aids digestion and can help with nausea and morning sickness.

- **Garlic.** This potent herb acts as a natural antibiotic. There is also evidence suggesting that garlic can help prevent heart disease.

- **Rosemary.** A cold and flu fighter that is also a natural astringent.

- **Cinnamon.** An ultrafabulous sugar substitute without sugar's side effects. Studies have also indicated that cinnamon may help lower cholesterol and blood-glucose levels.

- **Cayenne.** This warm spice helps to bring blood to the skin, giving you a healthy, rosy-cheeked look.

JUICE COUTURE

Freshly squeezed juice is beauty in a glass. It helps rid the body of toxins, brings more clarity to the mind, increases energy levels, and supports the immune system—all while feeding the skin essential vitamins from the inside out.

I try to eat at least 65 to 75 percent of my diet as raw fruits and vegetables. Fresh juice is a great way to get your daily raw veggie intake. During the cooking process, vegetables lose some nutrient value, including enzymes. Enzymes are important for many things, including building proteins in the skin. When you juice fruit and vegetables, the enzymes stay intact. Fresh juice is not only easy to make, it's also easy to digest. However, you can't *just* juice—you still need to eat whole fruits and veggies to get the benefits of their fiber content. I believe in a combination of eating steamed and raw vegetables as well as juicing them. Always try to buy organic fruits and vegetables. Conventional produce is sprayed with harmful pesticides, which are retained in the skins of many fruits and vegetables.

Juicing is also a great way for kids to eat their veggies. Put a cute curly straw in the glass and they will slurp it down in no time. Here are my three all-time favorite juice recipes.

Power Plant

Indoor air pollution can take a toll on your skin. But did you know that adding a little green to your home—literally—can detoxify the air? According to a NASA study, houseplants can remove as much as 87 percent of indoor pollutants, including things like benzene, formaldehyde, and trichloroethylene. Rubber plants, spider plants, bamboo, and peace lilies are all highly effective choices to help maintain healthy air at home—and a glowing complexion.

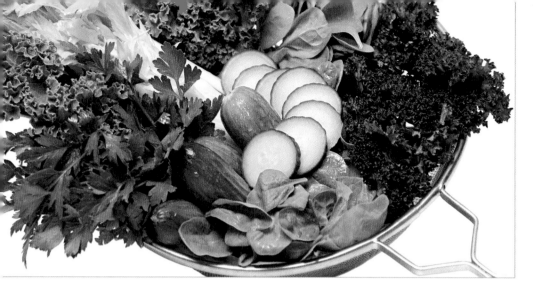

ALL GREEN

I was first introduced to this magic concoction when I was living in New York City. On my way to work, I would hop off the subway and stop by a local health food store that made fresh juices. Three times a week, I'd pick up a small-size juice blend called the "All Green," which consisted of green vegetables like kale, celery, cucumber, and spinach. After a month or so went by, my friends started to notice and comment on how vibrant and glowing my skin looked! I have to warn you, though, that great complexion comes at a price. The All Green isn't the tastiest or the most attractive beverage you'll ever find. But while it might not be pretty, you will *be if you drink this concoction several times a week!*

A handful of organic parsley

A handful of organic spinach

1 organic kale leaf

½ medium-size organic cucumber

4 or 5 stalks of organic celery

Put all ingredients through a vegetable juicer. Note: This drink tastes strong. You can add the juice of half of an organic lemon to lessen the potency.

(One 12-ounce serving)

BERRY BLAST

Berries are some of the best fruits you can eat because they are low in sugar and high in antioxidants and nutrients. When I need a quick pick-me-up on a hot summer day, there's nothing more refreshing than this delicious organic berry smoothie. If you're feeling sluggish, try my Berry Blast and you will be alert and energized in no time.

¼ cup organic raspberries

¼ cup organic strawberries

¼ cup organic blueberries

¼ cup organic blackberries

1 heaping Tbsp organic goji berries

2 cups almond milk

Put all of the ingredients into a blender and blend until smooth. Note: You can substitute soy or rice milk for the almond milk. You can also substitute organic frozen berries for fresh. They contain the same nutrient content and can be a convenient option when berries are out of season in your area.

(One 12-ounce serving)

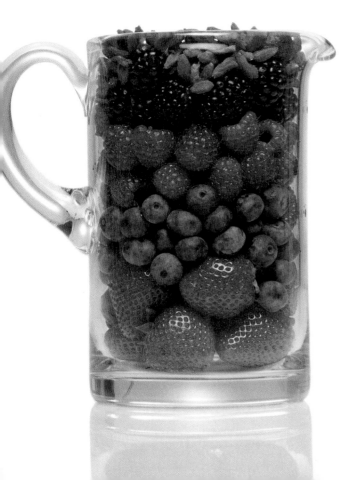

IMMUNE ZOOM

During the cold winter months, germs seem to fly around like crazy. Whenever I feel the signs of a cold coming on, I immediately make my Immune Zoom. It's filled with vitamin C and ginger, which are known to alleviate cold and flu symptoms. Did you know that a serving of strawberries contains more vitamin C than an orange? That's right. So with ginger, oranges, lemon, and strawberries, this immune booster will keep you from sneezing all winter long.

    5   medium-size organic oranges, peeled
    ½   oz fresh gingerroot, peeled and roughly chopped
    ½   organic lemon
4 or 5 organic frozen strawberries

Put the peeled oranges and ginger through a juicer. Squeeze the lemon juice into the mixture. Pour the contents into a blender. Add frozen strawberries and then blend until the berries are fully broken down.

(One 12-ounce serving)

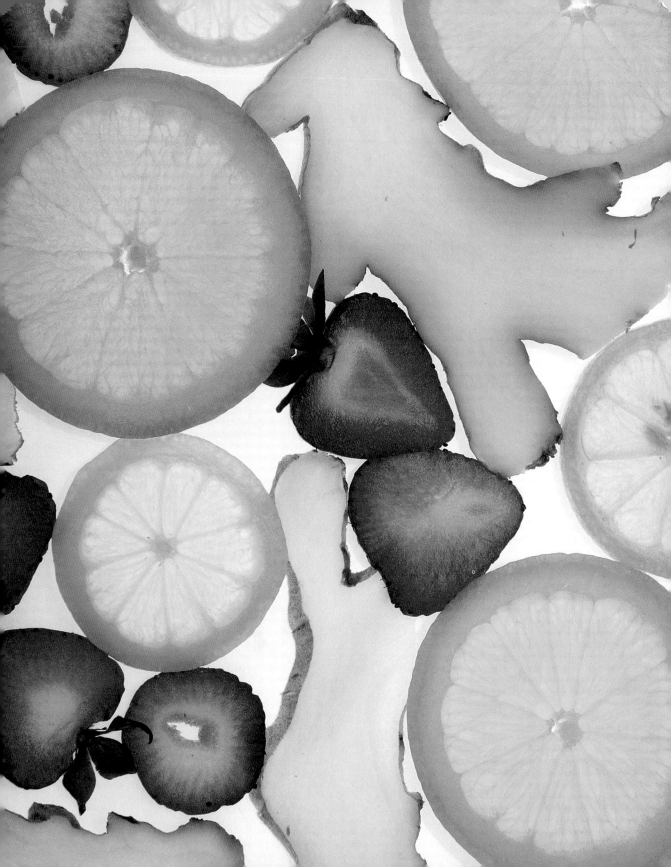

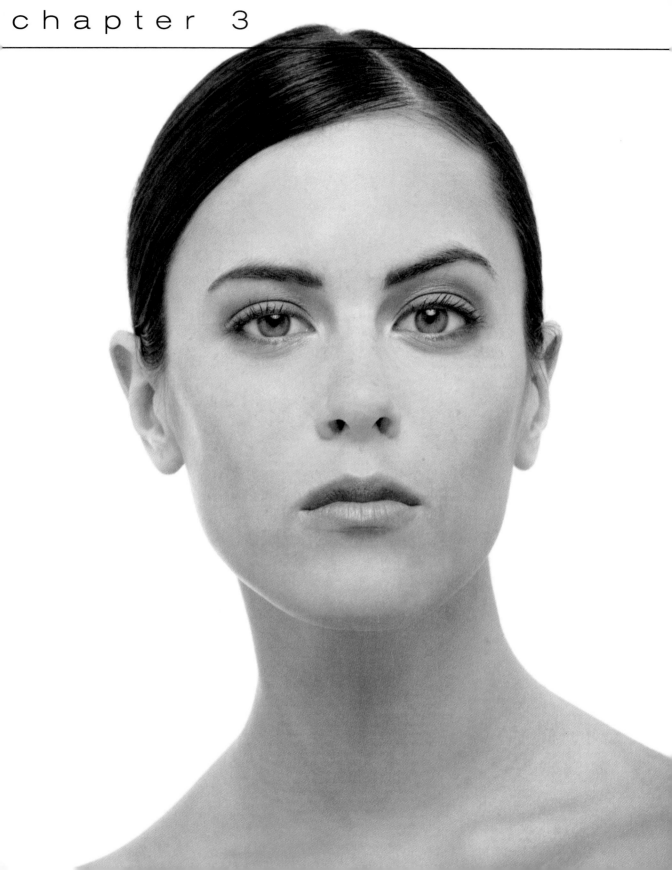

chapter 3

SKIN DEEP

Nothing makes a woman feel more confident than healthy, vibrant skin. But these days it has become more and more difficult to maintain a good complexion. Air pollution, car fumes, cigarette smoke, dust, and exposure to the sun are just a few of the everyday hazards that can take a toll on our skin. An unhealthy skin environment can even bring on eczema, which is a condition that results in patches of red, dry, irritated skin. If you have sensitive skin like I do, dealing with the toxins of the world is a battle you could use some help fighting. In Chapter 2, we discussed how to nourish your skin from the inside out. Now it's time to learn how to protect your skin from the outside in.

Many women use cleansers, toners, moisturizers, and masks to soothe their skin after its daily assault. But many of the skin products available at your local pharmacy are full of harsh, synthetic chemicals. Eco-friendly skin products are typically much gentler on your skin. My philosophy has always been that the simpler the ingredients, the healthier the skin. But before we discuss which eco-friendly beauty products you should use on your face, I want to share my four steps to maintaining beautiful skin:

1. Identify your skin type.

2. Treat your skin according to your skin type.

3. Commit to using eco-friendly skin-care products.

4. Start a daily skin-care regimen and be consistent.

It's crucial to know your own skin type so that you can begin to protect yourself from the very things that cause it to age. It's also important to know your skin type in order to take the necessary precautions to guard against various diseases, including skin cancer. But it's not always easy to know what type of skin you really have—sometimes it may seem dry, then it's oily, and breakouts can come and go. Here is my skin-type overview. See which type you are.

SKIN TYPES: 101

Normal skin. If your skin is neither oily nor dry, you have normal skin. You don't have flaky areas or greasy patches. Your skin has an even tone and a smooth texture. You rarely suffer from breakouts and your pores are an average size and never noticeably large. Your skin is also rarely irritated. Normal skin is the easiest type of skin to live with, but you need to take care of it. Neglecting your skin will lead to fine lines and wrinkles.

Oily skin. You have oily skin if you suffer from acne or have noticeably large pores or "shiny" skin. The oil glands in your skin are overactive and produce more oil than needed. This increased oil can cause breakouts and blackheads. This skin type sometimes looks coarse. Teenagers tend to have oily skin, but it usually becomes dryer with age. Pregnancy or menopause can also bring on oily skin.

Dry skin. If your skin often feels tight after you wash your face, you probably have dry skin. You may have breakouts, and you probably have some redness. Chapping and cracking are also signs of very dry or dehydrated skin. Dry skin has the opposite problem of oily skin—the oil glands do not supply enough lubrication and the skin ends up looking and feeling dry.

Combination skin. If you have oily skin on some parts of your face and dry skin on others, you have combination skin. You tend to be oily on the forehead, nose, and chin, and dry around the cheek and eye areas. Combination skin happens over time; changes are due to fluctuations in the seasons, your stress level, the environment, and your age.

TREATING THE SKIN YOU'RE IN

Now that you've figured out what skin type you have, it's time to look at what products are best for you. Your skin is the canvas for any cosmetic application. That's why we want to make sure your complexion looks as clear and healthy as possible. The best way to do that is to use products that contain only natural ingredients with no added fragrances.

These products still have the power to cleanse, tone, exfoliate, and moisturize effectively. Your skin can literally go from dry and flaky to smooth and vibrant or from oily and acne-prone to clear and gorgeous in no time if you choose the products that work best for you.

In the pages that follow, I will show you which eco-friendly products are the most effective for your skin type, including everything you need for the four steps of daily skin care: cleansing, exfoliating, toning, and moisturizing. I've also included homemade recipes with ingredients you can find right in your own kitchen. You can't get any more natural than that!

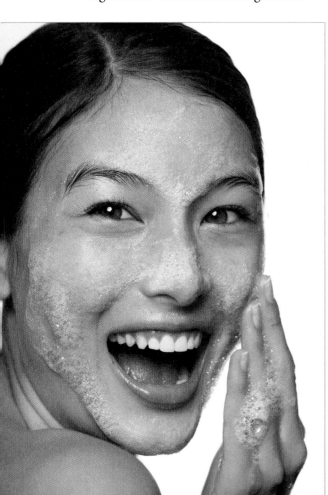

SOME LIKE IT HOT

Never wash your face with really hot water. While some beauty experts suggest that hot water cleans out your pores, the truth is that it can dehydrate your skin. Always use lukewarm water combined with a quality cleansing product.

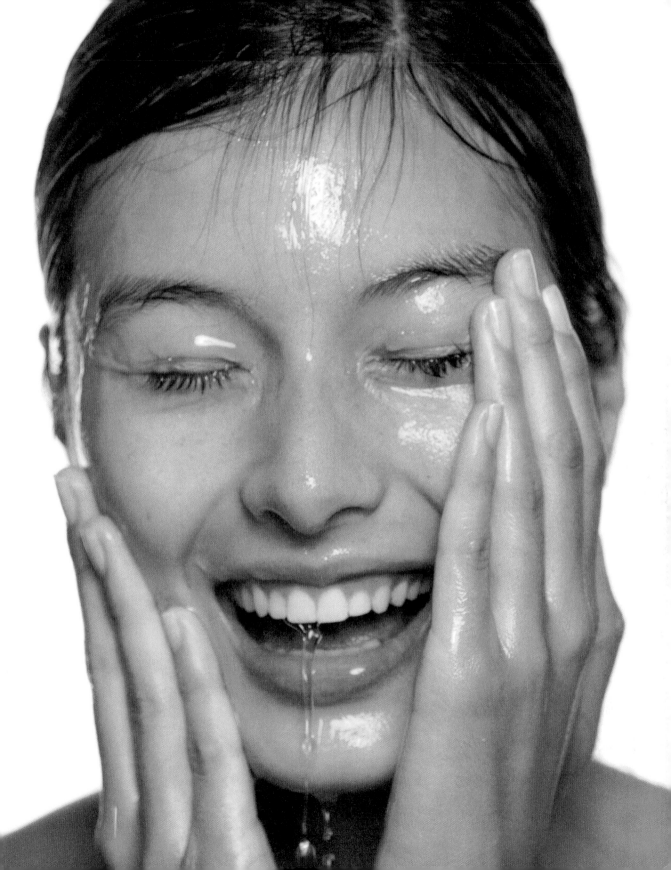

NORMAL SKIN

Cleanse

Wash your face twice a day with a very mild cleanser. This will keep your pores tight, but it won't dry out your skin. **Korres Magnolia** cleansing and moisturizing emulsion for the face is a fabulous, eco-friendly choice. It's rich in vegetable oils like wheat germ and almond—wonderful ingredients for normal skin. It also contains aloe and calendula to help retain moisture while it removes dirt and makeup with ease.

Do It Yourself

In my opinion, organic milk is the best natural cleanser for normal skin. In a small bowl, mix 2 tablespoons of organic whole milk with 1 teaspoon of sea salt. Then dab your face, avoiding the eye area, using an organic cotton ball. Let it dry for 2 minutes and then rinse off with lukewarm water.

Exfoliate

Normal skin should be exfoliated no more than twice a week. If you exfoliate too often your skin will produce more oils, thus leading to oily skin. Make sure you choose a gentle scrub with tiny grains. **Arcona Cranberry Gommage** is a wonderful product for normal skin. It unclogs and minimizes pores with ingredients like cranberry and raspberry enzymes while it prevents free-radical damage.

Do It Yourself

In a small bowl, mix together 2 teaspoons of uncooked, ground organic oatmeal and ¼ cup of plain organic yogurt. Apply directly to your face, using circular motions and avoiding the eye area. Rinse off with lukewarm water.

Tone

Toning the skin is an essential step in the cleansing process. It can really make a huge difference. It will remove any excess grease or makeup left on your face after washing. For your normal skin, choose a mild, alcohol-free toner. **Dr. Hauschka** facial toner hydrates the skin and minimizes pores.

Moisturize

Keeping your skin moisturized throughout the day is important. My suggestion is to moisturize two or three times daily. The best type of moisturizer for normal skin is a water-based cream with a hint of oil in it. **Aubrey Organics** facial cleansing lotion is a great option, as it tones and protects the skin with antioxidants like green tea and ginkgo and hydrates with oils like jojoba and aloe.

Do It Yourself

Bed of Roses: Rose water is a great natural toner for normal skin. It will leave your face feeling fresh and hydrated as it simultaneously stimulates the skin. And it's easy to make. Rinse 10 rosebuds and put them in a cup. Boil 1¼ cups of water. Pour the water over the rosebuds and cover the cup. Let it stand for about 20 minutes. Remove the cover, let the water cool, and strain out the roses. Pour the rose water into a small spray bottle and spritz it on your face. Keep refrigerated for up to 3 days.

OILY SKIN

Cleanse

The good news is that oily skin is less prone to fine lines and wrinkles than other skin types are. The bad news is that it's more prone to breakouts and acne. Stick with a cleanser that is water-based and oil free. One I highly recommend is **Miessence Certified Organic** purifying skin cleanser. It contains fresh lemon peel oil to tighten the skin, as well as witch hazel and burdock to keep the skin feeling soft without leaving it dry.

Exfoliate

Exfoliating is an important step in the daily regimen for your skin type. It will remove toxins and oil buildup and will allow your skin to breathe. This, in turn, will lead to fewer, or hopefully *no,* breakouts. Make sure to exfoliate two or three times a week after your breakouts have cleared completely. An excellent scrub for oily skin is **mod.skin labs Samurai Scrub Rice & Enzyme** face polish. With beneficial organic ingredients like aloe juice, vitamin E, green tea extract, cranberry extract, and mango butter, this exfoliating scrub will leave your skin looking and feeling amazing.

Do It Yourself

Mix the juice of one organic lemon and half of a pureed organic cucumber in a small bowl. Apply the mix to your face with a cotton ball, avoiding the eye area. Thoroughly rinse with cold water. It will cool and gently tighten your skin, leaving it fresh for hours.

Do It Yourself

A great homemade scrub that not only removes dead skin cells but also leaves your skin feeling soft and clean can be made from a very simple mix of lemon juice and sea salt. In a small bowl, combine ¼ cup of freshly squeezed organic lemon juice and ½ cup of sea salt until the two ingredients turn into a paste. Scrub your face with it, avoiding your eyes. Rinse completely with cool water. Use this scrub up to twice a week.

Tone

Using a toner every day after cleansing is an essential step for oily skin. A toner that works like a dream is **Aubrey Organics Blue Green Algae** facial toner. It clears away excess oil and calms and soothes the skin with organic and all-natural ingredients like balm mint, burdock root, elder flower, and lavender water.

Moisturize

Even oily skin needs to be moisturized at least twice a day. Use a lotion or a gel rather than a cream. The lighter the moisturizer the better for oily skin. **Arcona Magic White Ice** is a great hydrating gel. It's very light, but it moisturizes deeply and clarifies your skin with ingredients like cranberry and grapefruit extract.

Do It Yourself

Tomato juice is wonderful to use in a natural toner because it will reduce the size of your pores. In a bowl, mix ¼ cup of organic tomato juice and 1 cup of organic watermelon juice. Apply with a cotton ball, avoiding your eyes. This mixture will leave your skin feeling oh so fresh!

DRY SKIN

Cleanse

If you have dry skin you probably already know how difficult it can be to find products that work for you. Harsh chemicals, heavy fragrances, and cleansers containing alcohol will usually make your skin even drier. Cleansing milks and cream cleansers are a good choice for you, because they contain more moisture than most gels or soaps. Do *not* cleanse your skin more than twice a day. **Stella McCartney Gentle Cleansing Milk** from her Care line of organic cosmetics is a mild cleanser that removes impurities while soothing and comforting the skin. It contains sesame seed oil to help rebuild the skin's barrier and protect it from drying.

Exfoliate

Dry-skinned folks should exfoliate less often than those with any other skin type. Once a week is plenty. A fabulous choice is **Aubrey Organics Jojoba Meal & Oatmeal** mask and scrub. It's deeply moisturizing and will gently clear dead skin away, leaving your skin smooth. It contains avocado oil and carrot oil to replenish lost moisture and nourish the skin.

Do It Yourself

In a bowl, mix ¼ cup of organic cream, ¼ cup of organic milk, and 2 tablespoons of dried chamomile flowers. Heat the mixture over a low flame for about 30 minutes (do not let the milk boil). Then, let it sit for an hour. Apply the mix using a cotton ball and rinse off. Your dry skin will feel soft and glowing!

Do It Yourself

You can make an excellent homemade scrub that works for very dry skin from almonds and mayonnaise. Grind half a handful of raw, organic almonds in a blender. Mix in ¼ teaspoon of mayonnaise. Scrub gently and leave on skin for about 10 minutes. Rinse off with water. Repeat once a week, or twice a week for extremely dry skin.

Tone

Unless your skin suffers from extreme dryness, toning your skin can be very beneficial—as long as you use a mild toner that doesn't contain alcohol. You should use toners that contain herbal extracts to calm the skin. Look for ingredients like chamomile, cucumber, or rose oil. **Ecco Bella Mist-On Toner** contains essential oils to maintain the natural pH balance of your skin while restoring its vitality.

Moisturize

Moisturizing your dry skin is the most important step in this regimen. Choose a moisturizer with care. It should contain essential oils that will soothe and protect your skin. **Aubrey Organics Rosa Mosqueta** rose hip moisturizing cream soothes and moisturizes with almond oil, organic aloe, and rose hip oil. It has a coconut fatty acid cream base that will protect your skin.

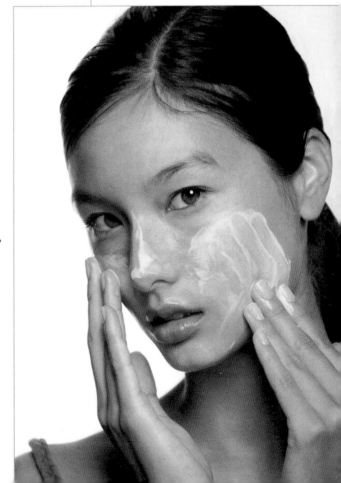

COMBINATION SKIN

Cleanse

If you have combination skin, you may find that when you wash your face, some areas feel tight while others look shiny. Wash your face with a mild and gentle water-based cleanser. **Korres Orange Blossom** cleansing and moisturizing emulsion is a great choice because it cleanses and moisturizes while it soothes inflammation of the oily part of the skin. It contains calendula, horse chestnut, and almond oil.

Do It Yourself

For combination skin, a yogurt cleanser can work wonders. Cleanse and exfoliate in one step by mixing 1 teaspoon of baking soda with 1 teaspoon of organic plain yogurt. Apply the mixture to your face and leave it on for 2 minutes. Then, gently massage into skin and rinse well with warm water. This cleanser works for your skin as it removes dead skin cells, cleans out the pores, and softens the dry areas of your face.

Exfoliate

People with this skin type should exfoliate about twice a week. Choose a scrub that purifies pores, while at the same time soothing the dry areas. **Arcona Golden Grain Gommage** purifies pores and soothes the skin with oatmeal and lemon extracts, leaving your skin feeling fresh and vibrant.

Do It Yourself

Mix 2 teaspoons of fine organic uncooked oatmeal and 1 teaspoon of baking soda. Combine the ingredients in a small bowl and add a touch of water to make a paste. Apply to your skin and rub gently in circular motions, avoiding your eyes. Rinse with lukewarm water and pat dry.

Tone

Toning your combination complexion is important, as it will help balance the pH of your skin and leave it more even and smooth. **Aubrey Organics Blue Green Algae** facial toner helps balance the complexion with all-natural herbs like peppermint leaf, calendula flowers, elder flower, and milk thistle.

Moisturize

Moisturizing combination skin will help balance and improve the skin's condition over time. Use a cream moisturizer that has a variety of different ingredients—such as sunflower oil and jojoba seed oil—for both dry and oily skin. **Miessence Balancing Moisturiser** is a good choice for your skin type. This product will hydrate and balance the dry and oily parts of your skin.

Do It Yourself

This homemade toner will hydrate and balance your skin. In a small bowl, mix 1 cup of water, 4 tablespoons of apple cider vinegar, 8 drops of rose oil, and 8 drops of chamomile oil. Use a cotton ball to apply to your face, avoiding your eyes.

AFTER-WORK ALL NATURAL BLISS

We all work hard to make a living. It's important to take a little time for yourself to decompress. A few times a week, save 20 minutes at the end of your day to take a nice, relaxing bath. Here is my three-step, at-home, eco-friendly program to achieve pure relaxation and rejuvenation.

Step 1

Light my fire. Light a candle to add some tranquility to your bathroom. These days, the best and most popular choice for the eco-conscious consumer are soy candles. Soy wax is non-toxic and made from soybeans, which are a renewable resource. Just like regular paraffin candles, soy candles come in various shapes, sizes, colors and scents. You can easily pick some up at your local Whole Foods Store or on the Internet.

Step 2

Soak your troubles away. Fill the tub with warm water and add an eco-friendly bath powder. **Sensatia Botanicals** (sensatia.com) offers fabulous bath powders in different varieties. Ingredients like unrefined sea salt, oatmeal, and tea tree oil will detoxify your body naturally. Simply add 2 tablespoons of the powder to your bathwater and relax.

Step 3 | **Smooth it out.** After your bath is complete, it's important to moisturize your entire body. **Desert Essence Organics** (desertessence.com) offers an entire line of lotions in many different scents that are 100% vegan as well as wheat and gluten free. I enjoy their **Vanilla Chai Hand and Body Lotion.** Rub the lotion it into your legs, arms, and shoulders. And don't forget your feet, especially your heels. I suggest trying their **Pistachio Foot Repair Cream.** It works wonders for dry feet.

A Cut Above the Rest

We can get pesky little cuts. And the smallest ones can hurt the most! The quickest way to heal cuts and scrapes is to stimulate cell production with a product like **Burt's Bees Res-Q Ointment** (burtsbees.com), which is a blend of the leaf and root of the comfrey plant. After cleansing your cut, simply apply a bit of the ointment twice a day and you will soon feel relief. This is a must-have for the "green" girl's first aid kit.

HERE COMES THE SUN

Many of my female friends say they haven't sunbathed in years and will never do it again. That's a good attitude to have, but women also need to realize that the sunbathing they did during their teen years can still cause damage. According to the Skin Cancer Founda-

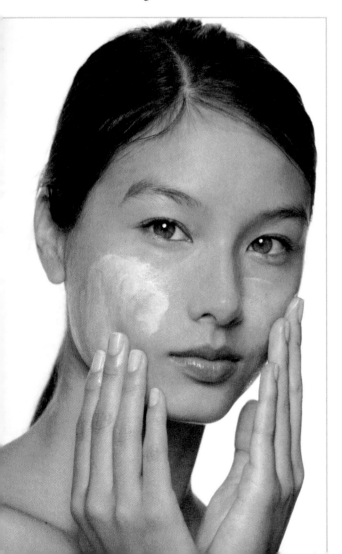

tion, the most common form of cancer in women ages 25 to 29 is, in fact, melanoma. Melanoma is a dangerous form of skin cancer that is brought on by UV rays from the sun and even from your local tanning booth. The initial signs of melanoma are physical changes to a mole—size, shape, or color. If you have spent considerable time in the sun, I suggest checking your skin once a month to look for any changes, and be sure to see your dermatologist every year for a skin cancer screening.

Unprotected time spent in the sun can also cause premature wrinkles and dark spots. In fact, sun exposure is considered by many doctors and scientists to be one of the biggest causes of skin aging, and it's almost impossible to avoid, especially if you live in a sunny place like I do. Recently, I was running late for an errand and left the house without putting on sunscreen. In my travels, I ran into a friend of mine on the street and we chatted for a bit. Time flew by and we wound up talking for approximately 20 minutes. The sun was behind me the entire time and when I got home, I realized the back of my neck was burned. All it took was 20 minutes! It amazes me how strong the sun is.

The very best way to protect yourself from the sun is to always—and I mean *always*—wear sunblock when you go outdoors. Applying a facial moisturizer with an SPF of at least 15 is the surest way to stay protected. It's also important to apply a body lotion with an SPF if your arms, legs, chest, or back are exposed. Also, remember to put sunscreen on the backs of your hands and the tops of your feet.

Some sunscreen brands can actually make matters worse because they may contain harmful synthetic chemicals, preservatives, and dyes. In fact, the ingredients in some conventional sunscreens can cause a plethora of skin allergies. When our skin is exposed to the sun our pores enlarge, and every product we put on our skin can be easily absorbed into our bodies. The good news is that there are many eco-friendly and oil-free options that will protect your skin and not clog your pores. Eco-friendly sunscreens are "protection plus." Not only do they protect you from harmful UV rays, but they also contain natural ingredients that *prevent* the signs of aging.

D-Day

The sun does offer *some* good things for us healthwise, like allowing us to absorb the vitally important vitamin D. However, instead of getting your vitamin D by frying on a beach blanket, I suggest adding it to your diet. Fatty fish like herring, albacore tuna, and salmon contain vitamin D. If your doctor approves, you should eat a fatty fish once a week.

Protection Plus

SPF FOR THE BODY

- Jason Natural Cosmetics Chemical Free sunblock, SPF 30+
- Aubrey Organics Natural Sun Green Tea protective sunscreen, SPF 25
- Santa Verde Aloe Vera Suncreen SPF 18

SPF FOR THE FACE

- Juice Beauty Mineral Sheer moisturizer (for all skin types), SPF 30
- Arcona Reozone full-spectrum sunscreen for face and body, SPF 20
- Kiss My Face Cell Mate 15, facial cream and sunscreen, SPF 15

Burn Notice

An itchy and hot sunburn is the *worst*. When it's a really bad case, it can make you feel like you want to jump out of your own skin. For fair-skinned folks, a sunburn can come from just 15 minutes spent unprotected in the sunshine. What's the best way to treat your skin after you do get sunburned? Time is undoubtedly the best medicine. But, when you feel uncomfortable and it hurts, it's nice to apply something cool and soothing to the skin so you can get some comfort and move the healing process along. Many women apply moisturizing creams, thinking they will

help. In fact, they actually make matters worse. Heavy creams trap in the heat and don't let the skin breathe, and they may contain alcohol or fragrances that will further irritate your very sensitive skin.

The best way to help the skin-repair process along is to use a simple remedy that takes advantage of natural skin soothers. Some of my favorite do-it-yourself recipes follow. They're easy to make, and you probably already have some of the ingredients in your pantry. However, before applying any remedy, the first crucial step is to cool down the skin. The best way to do that is to take a cool shower or bath. You can add 1 cup of oatmeal into the bath, which soothes the discomfort of a sunburn, or baking soda, which helps skin retain moisture. After bathing, I recommend wrapping an ice pack in a damp cloth and holding it over the sunburn.

Natural After-Sun Soothers

Lettuce wraps. Applying boiled iceberg lettuce water is a natural and effective sunburn remedy. After you boil the lettuce, turn off the heat and remove the lettuce from the pot of water. Put the water in the refrigerator to cool, then dip a soft, clean towel into the water and place it directly onto the trouble spots.

Alohhhhhh. Take a leaf from an aloe plant, break it in half, and apply the gel that oozes from it directly onto the burned area. Many health food stores carry fresh organic aloe leaves in the produce section, especially during the summer. If you can't find an aloe plant, use bottled 100 percent aloe vera gel that contains no added ingredients.

Cool as a cucumber. Organic cucumbers are not just good for reducing eye puffiness, they're also very effective for soothing sunburned skin. Apply thin cucumber slices directly onto your burned areas. It will help to ease the pain.

Tea time. If you fell asleep on the beach and your eyelids burned, I suggest using my tea bag remedy. Take two used black tea bags and put them in your freezer until they are cold. Then lie down, close your eyes, and place them on top of your eyelids for up to 20 minutes.

The Morning After

If you are looking for a quick fix for your under-eye-region after a night out on the town, I suggest using mod.skin lab's I.D. Zyne DMAE & Blue Green Algae. It goes on smoothly, will refresh the delicate under-eye skin, and improve the appearance of dark circles and fine lines.

THE ECO-GLAMOROUS FACIAL

When it comes to facials, there is only one place I go and recommend to my clients: the Arcona Studio (arcona.com). After my first facial at Arcona, my sensitive skin looked and felt amazing, with no hint of irritation or redness. I asked fabulous facialist-to-the-stars Chanel Jenae for her best skin-care tips.

What kind of negative effects have you observed from women using conventional cosmetics?

Oftentimes women overstrip and irritate their skin by using harsh chemicals like alpha hydroxy acid. Another big mistake women make is over-exfoliating, over-moisturizing, and using products that are too heavy for their skin. When these products are used, the skin cannot eliminate properly and the result is a lot of fatty deposits and congealed oil. When the skin can't utilize a really heavy product, it becomes clogged, over-soft, and the pores enlarge.

How often should someone get a facial?

It depends on a person's skin type, their goals, and what kind of shape their skin is in. However, the ideal situation for maintenance is to get a facial once a month. At minimum, every other month.

When you have oily skin, is it better to go to a facialist more or less often?

I think initially it is better to go more often because people with oily skin can benefit from professional peels and exfoliation. It will really jump-start their skin and get it to where they want it to be. Oftentimes, excess oil is due to something they are applying to their skin.

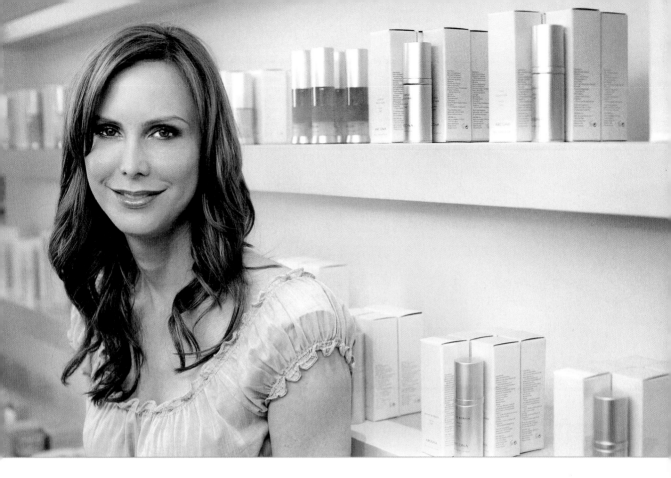

What are some things people can do in between facials to keep their skin healthy and glowing?

It's really about simplicity and maintaining a daily skin-care regimen. It is important to take care of your skin at night, no matter how tired you may be. We are exposed to dirt, pollution, and grime all day and the skin expels oils when you wear makeup. Night is the perfect time for the skin to regenerate.

Why do some experts say facials are bad for your skin?

People may go to facialists who are overzealous with extractions or who perform procedures they don't have the training to do. Sometimes people get a treatment and they are really marked up for days. Clients should be able to go to a facialist and not only feel really great, but also look really great when they leave.

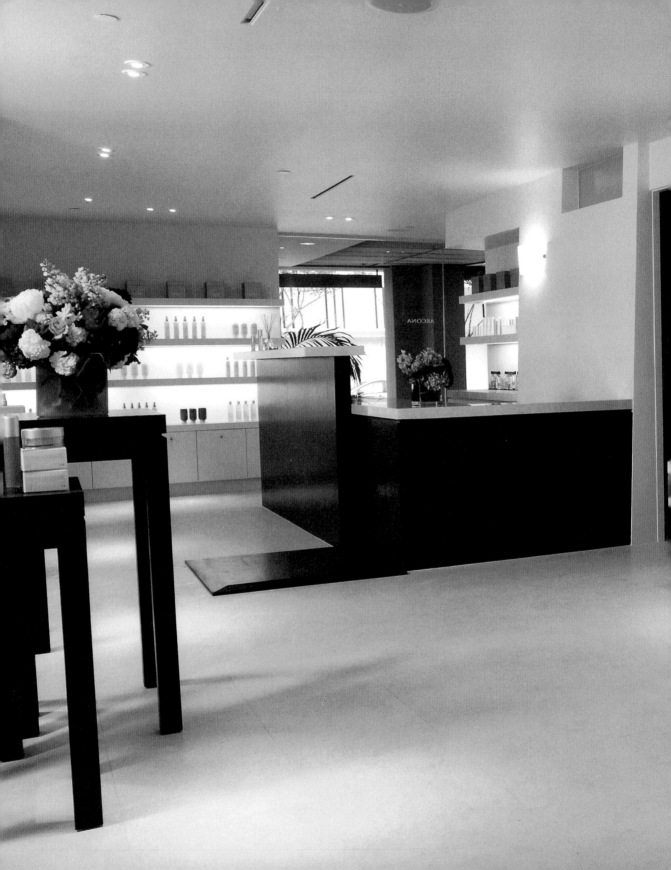

If someone is looking for a facialist, what questions should they ask before they surrender their face to them?

You need to do your homework just like you would when you are looking for a doctor, hairstylist, or makeup artist. It's important to get referrals—ask someone with great skin where they get facials. When you find an esthetician, ask them about their education. Is the place clean? Do they use gloves during the treatment, especially during extractions?

Chanel's Quick Tips to Beautiful Skin

- Drink water.
- Eat a lot of green foods, as well as foods that detoxify and nourish.
- Protect skin from the sun.
- Perform daily maintenance on your skin.
- Be happy!

chapter 4

ECO-AP

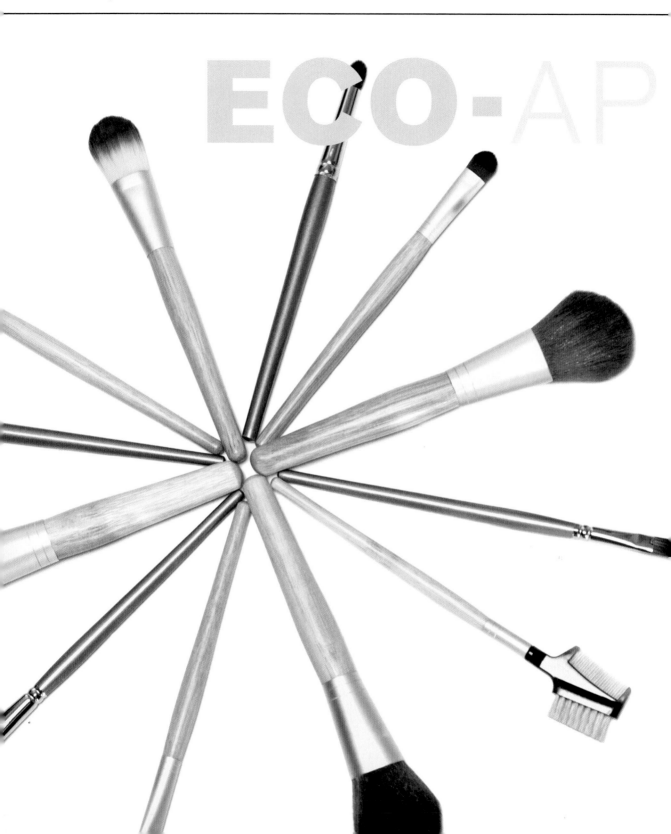

I've always loved the process of applying makeup. When I was 10 years old, I used to sneak into my mom's bathroom and play with all of her makeup. I had no clue what I was doing, but the experimentation, artistic expression, and transformation of my face got me hooked and made me want to become a professional makeup artist one day. As I got older, I took the time to learn more about how to apply makeup correctly, and in the process, I took the time to learn more about my own facial features. I also learned the importance of beauty maintenance. When you are able to do your own maintenance—like grooming your brows and taking care of your nails—you not only save money but, more importantly, you discover and better understand what makes you beautiful.

You also find out what does and doesn't work for you—a process of beauty trial and error. Don't be afraid to make a mistake during a makeup application. When you put on makeup, keep an open mind and be willing to take risks. Through the application process you will eventually find out what looks best on you.

In the previous chapters, we discussed the many eco-friendly cosmetics choices that are available and how they can benefit your skin; the foods and oils that can enhance your skin from the inside out; and the ways you can create a personalized daily skin-care regimen that will keep your skin healthy. In this chapter, I will help you understand how to accentuate your best facial features, explain easy techniques for beauty maintenance, and show you my tricks for applying a flawless face . . . or what I like to call "eco-application."

CLEAN CANVAS

Makeup application begins with a clean canvas: a combination of glowing, healthy, and clear skin, along with the appropriate shade of streak-free foundation and the right concealer. Once you've achieved this perfect base you're on your way to a truly eco-*beautiful* look.

I often see women making the common mistake of wearing way too much powder or the wrong shade of foundation. Or, when it's not blended properly, leaving them with a noticeably different color on their neck than on their face. Remember, the goal is to create a perfect canvas that looks as if

Throughout the next chapters, I've recommended some of my favorite products in a variety of price ranges. There is room for eco-beauty in every budget!

$ 1–25

$$ 26–39

$$$ 40 and higher

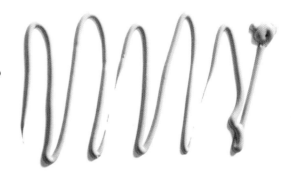

you're not wearing any makeup at all. And to do that, it's very important to pick the correct foundation for your skin coloring and blend it properly. Here are my step-by-step instructions for choosing and applying foundation.

Liquid Foundation and Tinted Moisturizer

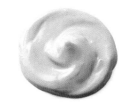

Liquid foundation is the most common form of foundation and is widely available. It works on pretty much any skin type, goes on smoothly, is very easy to blend, and provides excellent coverage. Tinted moisturizer is great as well, if you are looking for a sheer, natural look and you don't need as much coverage.

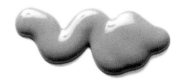

How to choose. Select a shade that is as close as possible to your skin tone. The best way to determine this is by applying a little foundation to your face in direct, natural sunlight. Take a look and keep trying different shades until you find the perfect match.

How to apply. Once you've found the right shade, apply the foundation to your cheeks, forehead, and chin. Then, using a makeup sponge or your fingers, blend it to even out the coverage. I prefer to use my fingers because the heat from your own body helps to blend the foundation

RECOMMENDED ECO-FRIENDLY LIQUID FOUNDATIONS

- Josie Maran Cosmetics tinted moisturizer $$
- Mineral Fusion Cosmetics sheer tint base $$
- Nvey Eco organic liquid foundation $$$
- Ecco Bella FlowerColor natural liquid foundation $
- Dr. Hauschka translucent makeup $$

into the skin even more effectively. Smooth out the foundation all over your face and down your neck as well as into your hairline for an even tone.

Cream Foundation

Cream foundation works best on dry skin because it has a thicker, heavier consistency. Also, eco-friendly cream foundations typically contain natural oils such as grape seed, sunflower, and jojoba, which can really benefit dry skin, especially during the cold and dry winter months. What I like about cream foundation is that it can be used as a concealer, as well. Using your cosmetics for more than one purpose not only saves you money, it saves you time and storage space, as well.

How to choose. Cream foundation works well if you are looking for a little bit more coverage. It goes on smoothly and is particularly good for women who have oily skin.

How to apply. Since cream foundation is thicker than liquid foundation, I

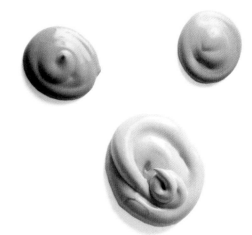

recommend dabbing your fingertips into the foundation, then lightly tapping it onto your face. Applying it this way, rather than with a sponge, gives you more control over how much you put on your face and makes it easier to blend. Because cream foundation can be thicker in some spots than others, make sure to blend it evenly over your face.

RECOMMENDED
ECO-FRIENDLY CREAM
FOUNDATIONS

- MyChelle cream foundation $
- Nvey Eco organic crème deluxe foundation $$$
- Monavé mineral cream foundation $

Mineral Foundation

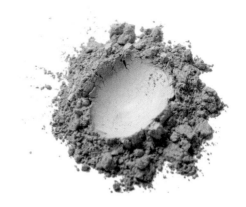

Mineral foundation works best for women with lighter skin tones. It can be difficult for women with darker skin tones to find a shade that works for them. Mineral foundation is an excellent choice for oily and acne-prone skin, as well as skin that is troubled by scarring, redness, or rosacea. It provides great coverage, but always remember to use a light hand. Too much can actually accentuate lines and wrinkles, and that's not what any of us want! A little bit goes a long way.

How to choose. Mineral foundation comes in a variety of forms—loose, pressed, and all-in-one brush applicators. The formulas for pressed and loose mineral foundations are often the same; but if you want a soft, air-brushed look, opt for loose foundation. Pressed foundation gives you a bit more coverage and lends a more natural look on top of liquid foundation than a regular pressed powder. The all-in-one brush applicator is a great on-the-go product for travel kits or quick touch-ups.

How to apply. Use an eco-friendly makeup brush such as the Lumiere **Cosmetics Baby Buki,** which is 100 percent synthetic, cruelty free, and vegan friendly. Dip the brush into the one loose mineral foundation shade that works best for your skin tone and gently dust

RECOMMENDED ECO-FRIENDLY MINERAL FOUNDATIONS

- Bare Escentuals bareMinerals SPF 15 foundation $
- Lumiere Cosmetics loose mineral foundation $
- Jane Iredale Amazing Base loose mineral foundation SPF 20 $$
- Monavé loose mineral foundation $

off the excess minerals (by blowing softly, or tapping the brush against the side of the container). Apply the foundation onto your cheeks, nose, chin, and forehead, using gentle circular motions.

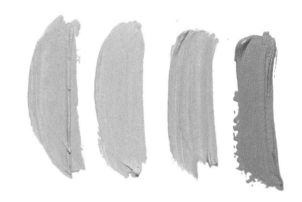

Concealer

Concealer picks up where foundation leaves off, evening out the skin tone and creating a flawless look. After you've applied your foundation, it's time to conceal any imperfections on your face such as redness, pimples, spots, or dark under-eye circles. Eco-friendly concealers will not only provide coverage, they'll also actually help to improve your skin. For instance, if you're covering up dark under-eye circles, eco-friendly products won't dry out this very delicate skin, and

they're free of dyes, talc, and starch—all things that can seriously irritate the eyes. If you are covering up a pimple, an eco-friendly concealer will not only help to hide it, but ingredients like tea tree oil will help it heal.

How to choose. I find that many women are afraid to use a concealer because they don't know how to apply it correctly or because it's difficult for them to find the right shade for their skin tone. To find the right shade, dab some concealer on your face in direct sunlight. If the concealer looks gray it means the shade is too light. If it shows up a little yellow it's too dark. A concealer that's the right shade should blend into your skin without showing up at all. When choosing an under-eye concealer, opt for one that has a bit more of a creamy texture and doesn't contain any tea tree oils, which will only dry out the eye area.

How to apply. Apply concealer to the under-eye area using a pointy concealer brush. I recommend Mineral Fusion's camouflage brush. A brush gives you more control than a sponge or your fingers would. Gently dip the brush in the concealer and brush it on. Apply the concealer on the dark areas under the eyes and gently brush it all the way up to the lash line. Next, apply concealer to the inner and outer corners of the eyes where there tend to be darker areas.

To cover up any unevenness or redness on your face, use the **EcoTools** concealer brush, which is 100 percent cruelty free and made of natural and recycled materials. Dot concealer on the pimple or the problem area using the brush or your fingertip, and remember to blend the edges so it looks even. Blending is the key for this makeup application! Don't forget to cover the inside of the nose bridge—a place where your skin can often look red. Don't apply more than two coats of concealer or it will begin to look caked-on and far too obvious. Remember, you are just concealing the problem area and you want it to look as natural as possible.

RECOMMENDED ECO-FRIENDLY CONCEALERS

- Dr. Hauschka liquid concealer $
- Jane Iredale Active Light under-eye concealer $
- Jane Iredale Circle\Delete under-eye concealer $$
- Josie Maran Cosmetics concealer $
- Sukicolor liquid formula concealer $$$
- Mineral Fusion Cosmetics concealer $$

Setting Powder

After you've finished applying foundation and concealer you need to *set* the makeup, so that the coverage lasts all day and doesn't rub off or crease. I suggest using a sheer, translucent powder for this step. I also like using a powder brush, as it will allow you to apply just a light amount of setting powder without overdoing it. This works for both pressed and loose powders.

How to choose. Look for a powder that contains ingredients like aloe vera and almond oil; this will benefit the skin *and* provide great coverage.

How to apply. When applying powder, gently brush the entire face using downward strokes. This technique will result in an even powder application. Throughout the day, you can touch up your makeup by applying some mineral powder using a small cosmetics puff on any shiny areas you want to blot, such as your forehead, chin, or nose.

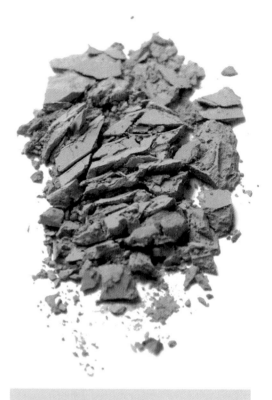

RECOMMENDED
ECO-FRIENDLY SETTING
POWDERS

- Ecco Bella FlowerColor face powder $
- Mineral Fusion Cosmetics setting powder $$
- Nvey Eco organic compact powder $$$
- Jane Iredale matte powder $$
- Josie Maran Cosmetics pressed powder $$

GET CHEEKY

Blush is a great go-to product that can quickly brighten up the face and help you look vibrant and healthy. If you are keeping long hours at work, stash a small blush compact in your purse for touch-ups when your skin starts to look a bit tired. Many women shy away from blush, but it can be your *secret* beauty weapon.

How to choose. Powder blush is the easiest form to blend over your foundation. The trick to choosing the right shade is to know what color your cheeks naturally flush. Look for all-natural brands that include antioxidants and anti-inflammatory ingredients. Make sure your blush is nontoxic, and fragrance and paraben free, because the pores on the cheeks can easily clog and cause irritation, pimples, and even rosacea. Here are some additional suggestions for choosing the perfect shade.

Ivory/Light Beige Skin Tone: Choose soft pink shades and tawny rose colors for a naturally rosy look.

Medium/Light Olive Skin Tone: Choose peach and apricot shades, which will instantly warm up your skin and give you a healthy glow.

Bronze/Dark Skin Tone: Choose dark, warm colors like cherry and cinnamon, which will give your skin a nice flush.

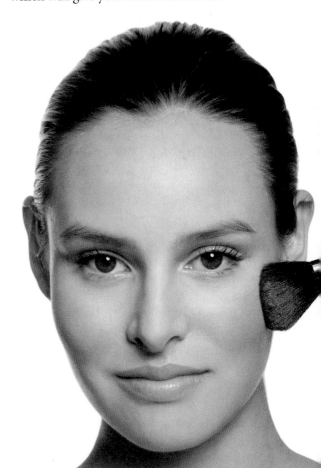

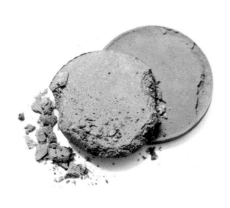
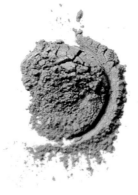
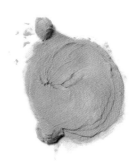

Black Skin Tone: Choose an intense color, such as deep red, red-brown, or plum.

How to apply. The apples of your cheeks are the best place to apply blush. Look in the mirror and smile. Apply blush to the portion of your cheeks that are raised using upward strokes. Make sure you invest in a good quality blush brush, such as the EcoTools blush brush.

Other Types of Blush

Loose minerals. Loose mineral blush works well for all skin types and skin tones. It gives you a sheer, natural look that even works well on top of a mineral foundation, liquid, or cream base.

Cream. Cream blush works very well on dry skin and mature skin. It gives you a soft, natural-looking glow. The best way to apply it is with your fingertips. Make sure to blend it well.

RECOMMENDED ECO-FRIENDLY POWDER BLUSHES

- Jane Iredale Pure-Pressed blush $$
- Nvey Eco organic powder blush $$
- Dr. Hauschka rouge powder $$

RECOMMENDED ECO-FRIENDLY MINERAL BLUSHES

- Lumiere Cosmetics mineral blush $
- Bare Escentuals bareMinerals All-Over face color $
- Monavé blush $

RECOMMENDED ECO-FRIENDLY CREAM BLUSHES

- Josie Maran Cosmetics cream blush $
- Sukicolor pure cream stain $$$
- Jane Iredale In Touch cream blush stick $$

BRONZED GLOW

Having a sun-kissed complexion can make a huge difference, especially during those cloudy winter months. While everyone else looks pale, a bronzer will warm up your face and help you look fresh. And when you have a sultry and sexy bronzed glow, your friends will ask which island you just got back from!

Applying bronzer is not the easiest technique to master. It can sometimes look uneven, streaky, and fake. But if applied correctly, bronzer will give you an eye-catching, natural glow. It's all about applying the right shade for your skin tone in the appropriate amount. Here are some basic guidelines.

HOW TO CHOOSE:

Fair Skin: Use a honey-colored bronzer.

Medium Skin: Use a gold-flecked or bronzy-colored bronzer.

Dark Skin: Use an amber shade of bronzer.

How to apply. First, make sure your face is dry and any moisturizer has been completely absorbed. Next, I recommend applying a little bit of translucent powder. This will help to prevent the bronzer from streaking due to moisture on your skin. It's best to apply bronzer in direct sunlight so you can easily detect any streaks. I recommend using a big, fluffy brush, like the EcoTools bamboo powder brush. Swirl the powder brush in the bronzer

RECOMMENDED ECO-FRIENDLY BRONZERS

- Dr. Hauschka bronzing powder $$
- Mineral Fusion Cosmetics bronzer $$
- Josie Maran Cosmetics bronzing powder $$
- Ecco Bella FlowerColor bronzing powder $
- Physicians Formula Organic wear 100% Natural Origin bronzer $

compact, dust off the excess on a tissue, and start applying the bronzer to your face. You should apply it only in the places where the sun would hit your face normally—the apples of your cheeks, your forehead, and your nose. Use soft circular motions when apply-ing. Start out with a little and then gradually work your way up to the desired shade. Remember to blend it well and make sure it is streak free. Lastly, don't forget to apply some bronzer to your chest and shoulders for the complete bronzed glow!

FIND YOUR FEATURES

We all have our own natural, God-given facial features. This is what makes us unique and gives us character. Some people have high cheekbones, other people have fuller lips or unique eye shapes or colors. Whatever your distinc-tive facial features may be, you need to find them, embrace them, and accentu-ate them. It's fun! Use my simple and effective makeup techniques and eco-friendly cosmetics suggestions to help bring out your one-of-a-kind beauty.

Eye-Catching

It has been said that the eyes are the "gateway to the soul." If that's the case, don't you think it's important to take extra special care of them? The skin around the eyes is the most sensitive and delicate area of your entire face. So when choosing eye makeup, the most impor-tant thing to remember is to pick prod-ucts that are gentle and nonabrasive. Eco-friendly makeup is the most gentle and effective makeup because it's free of preservatives and fragrances—which can irritate, cause puffiness, and dry out your eyes. The equation is simple: abrasive makeup + under-eye skin = fine lines and wrinkles.

Clients consistently ask me how they can bring out the color of their eyes. Well, there are many ways you can accentuate your eye color to really make it "pop" and help you get noticed. Every eye color can be high-lighted and enriched by using a complementary shade of eye shadow. Here are my top eco-friendly suggestions.

Brown Eyes

For Day: Plum, deep purples, and deep moss greens look fabulous on brown eyes for both day and night.

For Night: You can go black and dark smoky gray without looking too bold for a fabulous evening look.

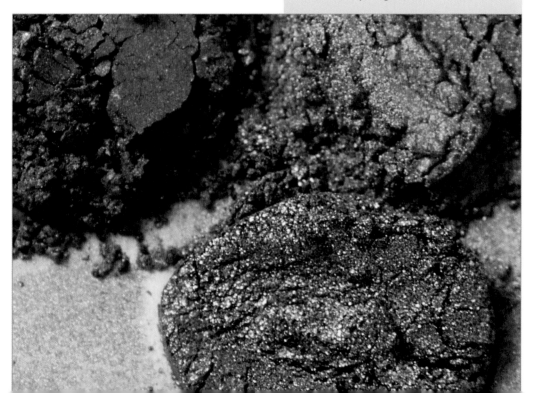

Blue Eyes

For Day: The blue in your eyes will pop with earth-tones, such as shades of gold and brown.

For Night: Metallic grays complement blue eyes well and are a perfect choice for an evening look.

RECOMMENDED ECO-FRIENDLY EYE SHADOWS

- Jane Iredale PurePressed triple eye shadow in Pecan Chocolate $$
- Bare Escentuals bareMinerals eye shadow in Camp $
- Dr. Hauschka eye shadow solo in Beach $
- Josie Maran Cosmetics eye shadow in Pewter $

Green Eyes

For Day: I adore the way golden beige looks against green eyes. It will make your eyes *shine*.

For Night: Dark browns and even purple shades are a fun choice for an evening makeup look.

RECOMMENDED ECO-FRIENDLY EYE SHADOWS

- Josie Maran Cosmetics eye shadow in Cinnamon $
- Neutrogena nourishing eye duo in Honey Nut $
- Josie Maran Cosmetics eye shadow in Cappuccino $
- Lumiere Cosmetics eye pigment in Light Plum $

Hazel Eyes

For Day: For more of a subtle look, pinks and golds will look refined and make your eyes appear lighter.

For Night: Metallic blue and navy will make your hazel eyes *really* stand out.

The Shape of Things

There are many different creative ways of applying eye shadow to enhance or correct the shape of your eyes. And it's simple. Just follow my tips below.

Wide-set eyes. To create the illusion that your eyes are set closer together, emphasize the inner corner of your eyes by applying eye shadow from the inner side of the upper lid and under the brow. Then, start applying a liner from the inner corner of the eye, and bring it out near the nose ridge. Last, apply a brow pencil to fill in your eyebrows, making sure the length of each brow is equal to the width of your eyes.

Almond-shaped eyes. Use a lighter shadow from the inner corner of the eye to the center and apply darker shadows to the outer corners. Make sure to blend well. Do not highlight the brow bone too much, as this will bring it more forward.

Small eyes. Don't use dark eye shadows or eyeliners. They will only make your eyes appear smaller. Instead, use lighter shadows on the eyelid, a slightly darker shade on the crease, and a highlighter on the brow bone.

Close-set eyes. Apply lighter colors to the inside corner of the eyes. This will push the eyes farther apart. Use darker shades on the outer corners.

Large eyes. To make your eyes appear smaller, apply a darker shadow on the lid and extend it to the crease. Avoid bright colors, as they will emphasize the fullness of your eyes.

Lashing Out

Most mascaras on the market contain artificial ingredients, preservatives, tar, and alcohol—all of which can do a number on your eyelashes. They will not only weigh down your lashes, but

Trick of the Trade

Create the illusion of longer lashes by positioning the mascara wand at the base of your lashes and rolling it horizontally as you glide it through the lashes. This will create long-lasting, full lashes.

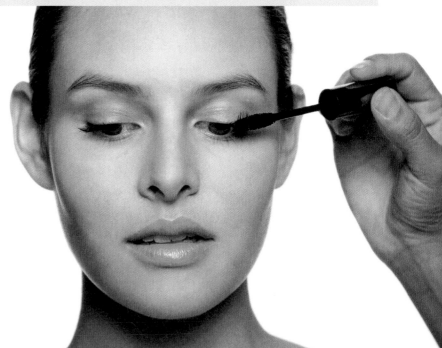

they will also make them weak. And a lot of women already have thin and brittle lashes due to hormonal changes or overuse of eyelash curlers. All-natural mascaras are packed with natural and beneficial ingredients, which will actually *improve* the quality of your lashes over time. So your lashes will look full and flowing, and they will also stay long and strong!

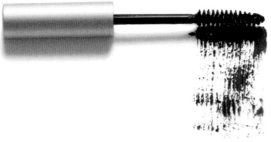

Just Browsing

Your eyebrows create a big impact, and perfectly maintained brows can make a noticeable difference in your appearance. They open up the eyes and make them look bigger, brighter, and bolder. However, the most common mistake that I see time and time again is the overpluck. Ladies, you must embrace your brow shape! Never make your brows thinner.

The premiere eco-friendly cosmetics choice for mascara is one that is made from minerals and plants. This will nourish, protect, and enhance your fragile lashes.

RECOMMENDED ECO-FRIENDLY MASCARAS

- Dr. Hauschka Volume mascara $
- Sukicolor Rich Pigment mascara $$
- Josie Maran Cosmetics mascara $
- Mineral Fusion Cosmetics lengthening mascara $

There's nothing natural looking about very thin brows. Naturally full brows, if you have them, complement your features much better. If you prefer to go to a salon for maintenance, stay away

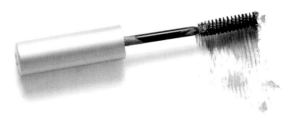

from wax and ask them to just clean up your brows with a tweezer and scissors.

The best time to tweeze is immediately after showering. It will be a lot less painful because the warm water and steam will have already opened up your pores and made the brow hair more manageable. Use a white eyebrow pencil to draw an outline of the desired shape. (Determine the best shape by using my pencil trick below.) Now you can just tweeze the hairs that are covered in white pencil.

If your brows are too thick and dense, a good way to soften them is to trim them, using a small pair of scissors. Just brush them up using the brow brush and

RECOMMENDED
ECO-FRIENDLY BROW TOOLS

- "Go Green" Mini Slant tweezer (tweezerman.com). This is a sleek and effective tweezer that actually gives back. What do I mean? Well, with every tweezer sold $1 is donated to the Arbor Day Foundation (arborday.org) and a new tree is planted. Now that's what I like to call a "tree-zer."

- EcoTools bamboo lash and brow groomer. This is a brush and comb combination made of synthetic bristles that are 100 percent cruelty free. The ferrule is even made from recycled aluminum.

Get in Shape

Don't know how to shape your brows and worried about the dreaded overpluck? Here's a great little trick to help you find the right brow shape for your face. Just browse (no pun intended) my three easy steps below.

1. Line an eye pencil vertically alongside your nose. This is where the brow should start.

2. Line the pencil diagonally from your nose across the iris of your eye. This is where the eyebrow arc should be.

3. Line the pencil by your nose and extend it to the outer corner of the eye. This is where the brow should end.

Shine a Light on Me

When we do our eyebrows or any other beauty task that requires good lighting, we are using energy. Choose compact fluorescent lightbulbs (CFLs) for your bathroom. They can use up to 80 percent less energy than regular incandescent bulbs and have a lifetime of 10,000 hours.

snip any stray hairs you see. Then, brush the brow hair down and snip any strays that go past the brow line.

Color Me Bad

Tinting your eyebrows or eyelashes is a big no-no. I *never* recommend it to any of my clients. Tints contain chemicals that are *not* eco-friendly and can be

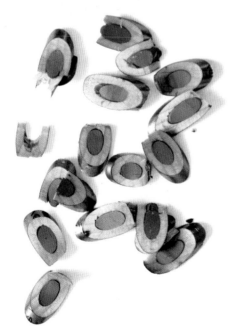

harmful to the delicate eye area. In fact, the FDA hasn't approved any of the color additives or tints used for dyeing eyelashes and brows. Furthermore, these color additives have been known to create side effects such as inflammation, swelling, redness, and infection. And these chemicals can go directly into your body through your pores.

On an aesthetic level, many women who tint their brows find it very hard to match their hair color. Tinted brows usually end up darker than desired, and the dye used is permanent. If you want to color your brows, I recommend using tinted brow gels, which come in different shades and they also wash out! There aren't many eco-friendly choices, but I recommend Jane Iredale Pure-Brow Colours.

GET READY TO RECYCLE

If there's just a little bit of lipstick left in the tube or some broken pieces of your favorite eye shadow in your makeup bag—don't throw them away. You can recycle them! As long as a cosmetic product is not expired, you can transform the last bits and pieces into something else new and exciting. And the small sizes are perfect for a travel kit. Here are some of my favorite recycling recipes.

Lip gloss. Do you have a little bit left of your signature lipstick? Make it your signature lip gloss in no time. Scoop out the remaining lipstick and melt by popping it in the microwave for a few seconds, then mix it with some clear lip gloss, let it cool, and store it in a small container. When it's ready, apply it to your lips using a lip brush.

Cream blush. Cream blush is a fabulous way to add color to your cheeks. Melt your leftover lipstick as above and after it's cooled, add some moisture to the cream by mixing in a couple drops of vitamin E oil. This will not only make the cream blush go on smoothly, but your skin will also benefit from the oil. Apply the cream blush using your fingers.

Cream eye shadow. We all know that eye shadows can easily break. It's even more frustrating when it's one of your favorite colors (not to mention if the

Eco-Beauty Sleep

We *all* need our beauty sleep. To help you get a proper rest, I recommend the **Natura Organic Sleep Mask** (dreamessentials.com). The inner part of the mask is made of certified organic cotton and the padding is made of organic Echo Wool. Don't forget to take it with you on your next airplane flight.

shade is discontinued). No need to worry any longer. Don't throw out your broken eye shadows when you can easily make them into cream eye shadows. Simply mash-up the broken eye shadow and mix it with an eco-friendly lip balm or shea butter, which contains anti-inflammatory properties, and store in a small container.

Tinted moisturizer. Foundations are one of the most expensive cosmetic products on the market. However, it's a must-have because it's used in almost every single makeup application. Recycling a little foundation here and there can make a difference. Use your favorite left-over liquid or cream foundation, mix it with an eco-friendly moisturizer. And store it in a small container. Now you have a recycled tinted moisturizer, which is a bit more sheer than regular foundation. This works quite well for a daytime makeup look.

LIP SERVICE

Here's an "all-consuming" thought for you. Experts say that the average woman will consume a pound of lipstick every year. That's right, a *pound*! So when choosing a lipstick it's vitally important to remember to look closely at the ingredients to make sure it doesn't contain any lead. Lead is a proven neurotoxin that can cause very serious health problems. Pregnant women should be extra cautious, as lead has been linked to miscarriage and infertility. Look for products that contain jojoba oil, shea butter, and other organic and natural ingredients instead. In the end, your lips will actually benefit from these ingredients. And that is the whole point of eco-friendly cosmetics—for your body and skin to actually improve through a simple application.

As a makeup artist I love having fun with lip colors. Lip color adds life to your face and can give you a completely different look depending on whether you go with a lighter shade or a darker shade. However, when choosing a color, it's important to keep your skin tone in mind. My rule of thumb is, the deeper your skin tone, the deeper the shade of lip color you can wear. Why? A dark lip color on a very fair woman can look way too dramatic. And on a darker-skinned woman, a dark lip color will show up better than a light lip color.

How to choose. Here are my guidelines for choosing the right lip color.

Fair Skin: Sheer pinks, light peach, nudes, and even cherry reds look best on fair skin.

Medium Skin: Rose and medium pinks and shades of wine look great on medium skin tones.

MAKE YOUR OWN ECO-FRIENDLY BEAUTY PRODUCTS

I've always adored cooking because not only do I find it therapeutic and cost effective, but I know exactly what is in the food I eat. The same goes for DIY beauty products. Of course, making your own makeup all the time is tough when you're busy, but if you have some time on your hands and you're feeling creative, I highly recommend giving it a try. It makes for a great weekend project on a rainy Saturday and it's a lot of fun! The steps are not difficult and you probably have many of the ingredients at home already.

MAKE YOUR OWN ECO-FRIENDLY
EYE MAKEUP REMOVER

When you're taking off your makeup, it's important to clean your skin properly. There are some great eco-friendly makeup removers in stores, but making your own eye makeup remover is not only good for the delicate skin around your eyes, it's also a great way to save money. The ingredients and steps are quite simple, and the result is clean and glowing skin.

What You Need

- 1 tablespoon of castor oil
- ⅛ cup of grapeseed oil

Mix together the castor and grapeseed oils in a small recyclable glass container. Shake well before using. Apply to your skin using a cotton pad or cotton ball and rinse with water.

MAKE YOUR OWN ECO-FRIENDLY
LIP BALM

Lip balm is one of those cosmetic products you should have on hand at all times. It's a necessity because nobody likes to look at or talk to chapped lips. It makes a difference between a good first impression and a bad one. People think that lip balm is just for cold weather climates, but it can be used all year around and protects your lips from all elements. And it's definitely not just for women. Lip balm has been called "the man's lipstick." Lip balm, like my favorite pen, is something that I tend to lose weekly. The remedy for this is to make your own.

What You Need

- 2 tablespoons of shea butter
- 4 tablespoons of olive oil
- 2 vitamin E capsules or vitamin E oil
- 4 drops of your favorite essential oil. (I recommend vanilla or peppermint because it will add a clean fresh scent to your lips.)

In a tall, heat-proof mug, mix the olive oil and the shea butter. Poke a hole in the vitamin E capsules and squeeze the liquid into the mix. Then, add the drops of essential oil. Fill up a small pot with boiling water and add the cup to create a hot water bath, which will melt the mixture gently. Next, pour the mixture into a small recyclable glass jar. Let it cool before using.

MAKE YOUR OWN ECO-FRIENDLY
BODY LOTION

Lotion is one of the most important beauty products to use daily. And there's nothing quite like the feeling of smooth lotion coating your skin after a refreshing shower or bath. Not only does it invigorate and pamper your skin, it also provides a layer of protection against chaffing, drying, and cracking. Below is my "Almond Joy" body lotion recipe—it smells great, but is not too obtrusive.

What You Need

- 1 organic egg yolk
- ½ cup almond oil
- ½ cup olive oil
- 2 tablespoons freshly squeezed organic lemon juice
- 1 teaspoon essential vanilla oil

In a bowl, whisk the egg yolk while adding the lemon juice. As you continue to beat the egg, add the almond and olive oils. When the mixture has thickened, add the essential vanilla oil. Pour into a glass jar and it's ready to use.

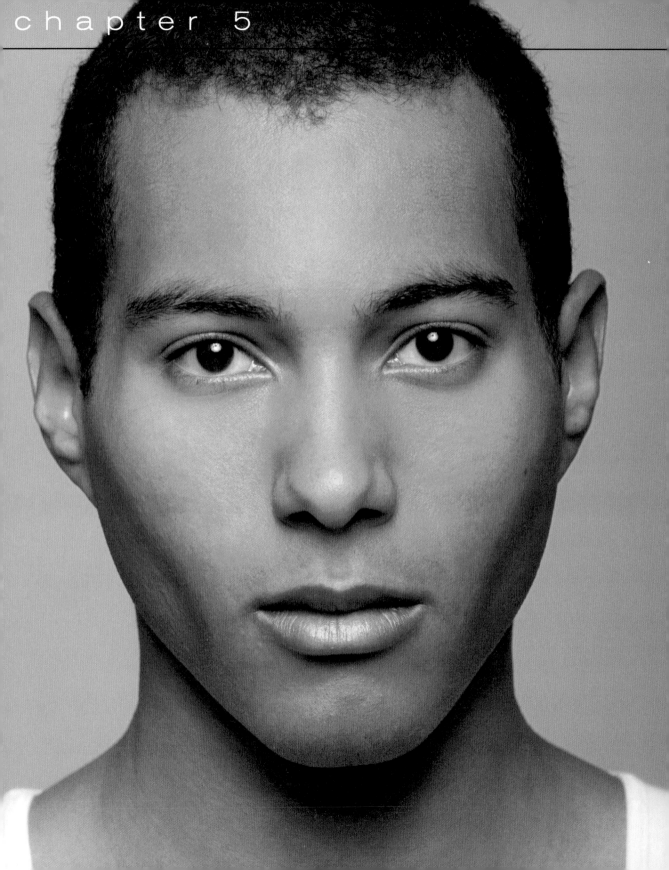

chapter 5

THE ALL-AROUND "GREEN" GUY

It's become much more socially acceptable—and even downright trendy—for men to take care of their appearance. From magazines like *GQ* and *Men's Health* to an ever-expanding personal care industry marketed to men, guys don't need to hide in a dark alley to apply moisturizer anymore. In fact, many women find a well-groomed man to be pretty sexy. Of course, it wasn't always like this. While I was growing up, I don't think I ever saw my father use moisturizer. *Exfoliate?* My dad only used four products: shampoo, shaving cream, deodorant, and toothpaste. And he used the same ones for 20 years! My mom and I found the simplicity of his daily grooming routine quite cute and refreshing. But these days, with the sun's rays growing more intense and countless environmental stresses wreaking havoc on your skin every day, shaving cream and toothpaste just aren't enough.

American men spend $4 billion a year—that's right, $4 *billion*—on skin-care products. There's now a wide range and variety of grooming products for men to choose from. There are even day spas that offer special facials just for male clients. Next time you get a manicure, count how many men you see inside the salon. Twenty-first-century men have broken the mold of what is deemed "manly."

With all of these services and products at their fingertips, it's just as important for every well-groomed guy to go green, too. After all, when a man takes pride in his appearance *and* pride in the environment around him, he's not metrosexual . . . he's *eco*-sexual!

ECO-SEXUAL

Since conventional grooming products for men are filled with many of the same harmful ingredients found in women's cosmetics, it's equally important for men to make eco-friendly choices. One common skin issue that many men experience is dry skin.

Dryness is more often than not a result of shaving almost every day with conventional shaving creams or soaps that contain harsh ingredients such as alcohol. Alcohol will dry out the skin and leave it looking red, flaky, and dry. In the long run, dry skin can lead to fine lines and wrinkles. Other common male skin problems include oily skin, clogged pores, breakouts, and blackheads—and they can all be fixed.

In this chapter, I will show men how to solve their skin problems by learning more about their own skin and how to take care of it. I will cover skin-care regimens, shaving techniques, and products for the ultimate eco-sexual man. Ladies, get your boyfriend, husband, or brother to read this chapter. They too can go green.

ALL SKIN IS *NOT* CREATED EQUAL

When it comes to their skin, men and women are *not* created equal. In fact, most men's skin is actually likely to age more gracefully than most women's skin. Why? One of the main reasons is that men's skin is firmer and made up of more collagen and elastin—two vital components in the fight against fine lines, wrinkles, and sagging skin. The difference is primarily due to hormones; men have more collagen because their bodies produce more testosterone. Women go through a lot of hormonal changes after menopause and their skin can suffer, especially if they are not eating well and using the right products. After menopause, female skin can lose elasticity and its ability to bounce back after damage.

A lot of my male friends have told me that in a pinch they sometimes use their girlfriend's or wife's beauty products, thinking it can't do any harm because their skin, after all, is less sensitive than a woman's. I quickly inform them that that's a *big* beauty myth. Overall, men's skin is surprisingly more sensitive than women's. Some research attributes this to the fact that men often spend more time outdoors, engaged in physical activity. Over time the sun, combined with environmental pollutants and toxins, can contribute to skin damage and increased sensitivity.

Men's skin has one major disadvantage compared with women's skin: shaving. If a woman cuts herself when she shaves her legs, she can just throw on a pair of pants. However, if a man nicks himself while shaving, there is no place to hide. Shaving can cause a variety of skin problems for men, such as rashes, bumps, ingrown hairs, and breakouts. And once the skin has broken out, shaving can spread bacteria to other parts of the face and cause the breakout to worsen. It can become a truly vicious cycle. Although men's skin is 20 percent more oily than women's skin, many men suffer from chronic dryness due to shaving with conventional products. Let's look a little more closely at how men can prevent dry, irritated, or broken-out skin by developing an eco-friendly shaving routine.

THE ECO-SHAVE

Every man is on the quest for the perfect shave. But how about the perfect environmentally friendly shave? Shaving is something most men do on an almost daily basis. So when you're doing something that frequently in your daily life, it's important to make sure that you're not harming the planet, or your face, in the process.

To achieve the closest and smoothest shave possible, a disposable razor is a better choice than the electric kind. There has been much debate over which one is better for the environment. My answer: Both can be eco-friendly if you choose the right products. It's true that disposable razors have been at the root of many environmental issues and concerns. The Environmental Protection Agency (EPA) estimates that 2 billion disposable razors end up in U.S. landfills every single year. And many razors are tested on animals. Thankfully, there are eco-friendly solutions to this problem.

One product I recommend is the **Preserve Triple Razor** (preserveproducts.com). Its recyclable handle is made of one solid piece of 100 percent recycled plastic, and 65 percent of that handle is actually recycled from Stonyfield Farm yogurt cups. (Pretty cool!) If you're concerned that this razor won't be as effective as the razor you're using now, think again. This razor is durable, flexible, and it pivots with the curves of the face. It also has a lubricated strip coated with moisturizing vitamin E and aloe.

Now, if you prefer to sport a five o'clock shadow or just like to use an electric razor, then I suggest the **Sol Shaver Solar Razor**. This electric razor is actually powered by solar energy. The only battery it takes is the big one up in the sky!

Selecting an Eco-Friendly Shaving Cream

Choosing the right shaving cream is just as important as selecting the proper shaving razor. A top-quality eco-friendly shaving cream will do wonders for the texture of your skin and will make your shaving experience smoother . . . literally!

When a man shaves his face the pores of his skin become enlarged and exposed. Not only can conventional shaving cream get into these open pores and cause breakouts and irritation, but the chemicals in that cream can directly enter the bloodstream. This is not a good thing. I highly recommend staying far away from aerosol-dispensed shaving products. Although chlorofluorocarbons (CFCs)—the propellant originally used to force a cream or gel out of a can—are now banned in the

United States, these products now use liquid petroleum gas, which still contributes to global warming. Furthermore, when you use aerosol creams you get more air than cream. And in order to achieve that fluffy white foam, hydrogenated fats are added to the formulation. I suggest you look for shaving creams that come in a squeeze bottle, manufactured by companies that do not test on animals and use only natural, plant-based ingredients. Here are three eco-friendly favorites.

- **Kiss My Face Fragrance Free Moisture Shave** (kissmyface.com): This shaving cream contains peppermint to cool the skin as well as aloe vera, coconut oil, and olive oil to assist with healing.

- **Weleda shaving cream** (usa.weleda. com): This is an extremely nourishing cream, with rich ingredients like goat's milk and almond extract. This cream does contain fragrance, but it's derived from natural essential oils.

- **Jason 6-in-1 Beard and Skin Therapy shaving lotion** (jason-natural. com): This will cleanse and condition your skin with vital ingredients like certified organic aloe vera gel. It is also pH balanced.

It's also important to be conscious of marketing slogans on men's grooming products. One popular claim that many conventional shaving cream products boast on their labels is "Dermatologist Approved." But this does not mean the product is eco-friendly or contains

Hair-Raising Experience

Years ago, actor/activist Woody Harrelson protested against Gillette. Along with PETA, Harrelson boycotted the company for its practice of testing on animals. Since then, Gillette has cleaned up their act and they no longer use any laboratory animals to test their products.

Lather Up If It Contains:

Aloe vera

Avocado oil

Calendula

Chamomile

Citrus seed extract

Distilled water

Green tea

Echinacea

Rosemary

Shea butter

Vitamin E oil

Steer Clear If It Contains:

Benzocaine

DEA (Diethanolamine)

Isobutane

Menthol

Petroleum

Propylene glycol

Sodium lauryl sulfate

Stearic acid

TEA (Triethanolamine)

natural ingredients. Instead, look for slogans like "Cruelty Free," "Soap Free," and "Propellant Free." The best part about eco-friendly products is that you *don't* have to take the bad with the good. You just take the good ingredients and reap all of the fabulous benefits for your skin. When choosing shaving cream, it's always important to read the list of ingredients. The above chart is a cheat sheet of the best and worst you can expect to find on shaving cream labels.

The Perfect Eco-Friendly Shave

Pre-shave. Exfoliating is the first step to getting a close shave. I don't recommend exfoliating every day because shaving already scrapes away dead skin. But twice a week, while you are taking a warm shower, I suggest using a mild eco-friendly scrub. It will remove dead skin cells and also bring the hair to the surface of the skin, which will help you avoid ingrown hairs. An exfoliator that I recommend is the **Aguacate & Co. Facial Exfoliating Crème** (aguacateandco.com). This product is infused with jojoba oil; it scrubs away damaged surface cells and moisturizes the skin.

The very best time to shave is when you have just stepped out of a warm shower. This is when the skin and beard are at their softest and

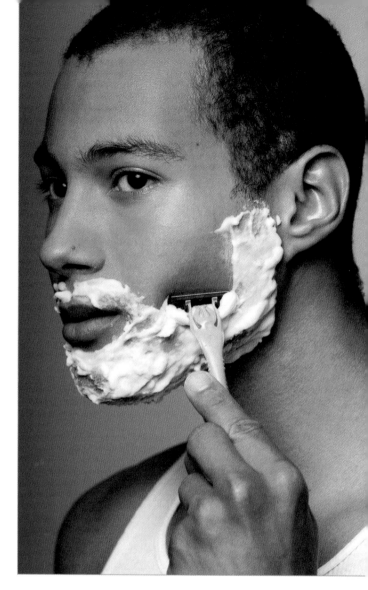

Da Balm!

Men want clear, smooth skin after a shave. The post-shave process is crucial to avoiding razor bumps and irritation. Use a natural aftershave, such as Aveda Men After-Shave Balm (aveda.com), which gives your skin comfort with aloe and chamomile extract. This alcohol-free product even helps to protect your skin by retaining water. This balm is da bomb!

easiest to shave. Rub some eco-friendly shaving cream in your hands and then apply it to your beard. Leave it on your face for about 5 minutes prior to shaving. At this point, instead of filling up the sink and leaving the tap running (a colossal waste of water), try filling up a small bowl with warm water and another small bowl with cold water. You'll use the warm water to clean the razor in between strokes and the cold water to rinse your face when you've finished shaving.

The shave. After you have left the cream on for approximately 5 minutes, you can begin shaving. Make sure you use a brand-new razor. (Previously used razors often contain accumulated bacteria and may cause breakouts and razor burn.) By now you probably know where your problem areas are—the parts of your face that are harder to shave or more prone to irritation. I suggest shaving these areas last so that they have more time to soften from the shaving cream. Plus, the blade of your razor will be

duller by the time it hits these sensitive areas.

Make sure you're not shaving too hard—there's no need to press down on the razor. If you have followed the steps recommended so far, the razor should glide over your face. Remember to shave in the direction the hair grows. This will minimize your chances of getting those pesky ingrown hairs. After every couple of strokes, rinse the razor in the bowl of warm water.

Post-shave. Once you have finished shaving your face, there's

Give Me a Break

Once a week give your skin a break from shaving cream by using organic olive oil. This essential oil has anti-inflammatory properties and many agree it can give an even closer shave than shaving cream. Just put a little bit of olive oil in your palm, rub your hands together a couple of times, and apply directly to your facial hair. You will be *amazed* at how easily the blade glides over your skin.

still another important step. The post-shave process is just as important as the pre-shave and the shave itself. First splash your face with the cold water from the second bowl. This will help to close the pores and tighten the skin, as well as wash off any leftover shaving cream. Then, pat (don't rub) your face dry with a clean towel. It's very important to use a clean towel on freshly shaved, sensitive skin. If, for example, you've wiped your hands on the bathroom towel after applying a hair product and then you use that towel to wipe your face, you could wind up with irritation or breakouts. Once your face is dry, apply an all-natural aftershave. Put

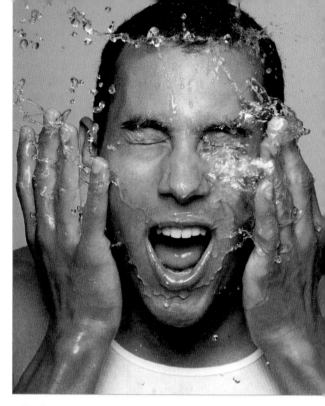

a little in the palm of your hand, rub your hands together, and then pat your face and neck. After you have applied the aftershave it's important to moisturize. More on that step next.

A Healthy Head of Hair

The ingredients in conventional hairstyling products, shampoos, and conditioners can damage men's hair and make the scalp dry and flaky. Eco-friendly hair products are made with natural oils (like tea tree and hemp seed) that will keep your hair from breaking and give it a healthy sheen. Also, consuming foods like beans, dark green veggies, and walnuts regularly will further strengthen your hair.

A DAILY DOSE OF ECO

Daily skin-care regimens aren't just for women. Men's skin can change dramatically for the better if you take just a couple of easy steps in the morning and at night, and if you use eco-friendly products that work for your specific skin type.

Keeping your skin clean is step *numero uno.* The daily cleansing process is extremely important for men no matter what skin type you have. It will wash away dirt, bacteria, and those pesky oily residues. Moisturizing your skin after shaving in the morning and again before bed will help make your skin feel soft and smooth. Always choose an alcohol-free moisturizer that contains natural oils and vitamins to moisturize your skin naturally.

Most men like to keep their daily routine simple, so I am going to offer skin regimens for men that are eco-friendly and effective, but not too elaborate. A little goes a long way, fellas. First step is to go to Chapter 3 and read "Skin Types: 101" to find out what skin type you have (yes, that chapter applies to you, too). Once you know your skin type, follow one of the regimens below and I promise you will be surprised at the change in your skin.

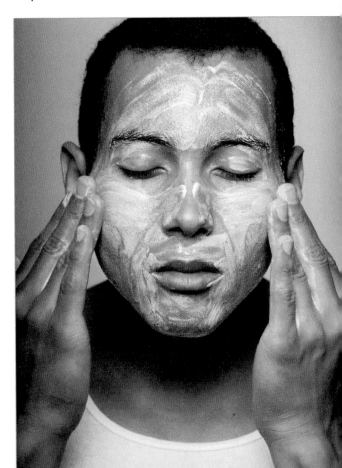

OILY SKIN

Cleanse

Cleansing your oily skin is important because it will reduce pores and blackheads. **Aubrey Organics Men's Stock** basic cleansing bar contains menthol to keep your face feeling fresh and cool and organic shea butter and sunflower oil to leave your skin feeling soft and smooth without overdrying.

Moisturize

Moisturize your skin twice daily (morning and night), but choose a moisturizer that is lightweight and not too thick or creamy. **Aubrey Organics Men's Stock** daily moisturizer contains flaxseed lignan extract, which helps balance oil production and won't clog pores, so it's perfect for oily skin.

NORMAL SKIN

Cleanse

Wash your face with a soap that is not drying and contains natural oils that gently wash away any dirt. **Burt's Bees Natural Skin Care for Men** bar soap is an excellent choice, as it contains bergamot fruit oil and rosemary leaf oil to keep the skin feeling fresh.

Moisturize

A hydrator that works well for normal skin and helps to keep it in good balance is **Arcona Cool Zone** daily facial hydrator. It contains EGF (epidermal growth factor) and will strengthen the elasticity of the skin.

DRY SKIN

Cleanse

Use a cleanser that soothes and heals the skin and contains natural oils to prevent your skin from becoming dry. **Arcona Kiwi Cream** bar is especially made for sensitive and dry skin and it is infused with vitamins.

Moisturize

Choose a moisturizing cream rather than a lotion to get a deep moisturizing effect. Opt for a cream with natural oils, but one that isn't too greasy. **Lavera Men Care** moisturizing face cream works great, as it contains vitamins and oils that penetrate the skin, leaving it soft and smooth.

THE OUTDOORSMAN

Whether you're on the golf course, washing your car, or playing a game of pickup basketball, the sun and all of its dangerous UV rays are shining down on your body the entire time.

With so much time spent outdoors and the dangers of skin cancer ever present, why do men continue to forget to apply sunscreen on a daily basis? For some reason even my most cautious male friends neglect to apply sunscreen. It's important to apply a light sunscreen every day—not just when you're on a boat or lying on the beach. And, as discussed in Chapter 3, conventional sunscreens contain ingredients that can cause a plethora of skin allergies. Before I recommend specific products, here are some important tips to remember before heading into the great outdoors (see box at right).

SUNSCREEN TIPS FOR MEN

- Apply it 20 minutes prior to heading outside. This way it will have time to dry and be absorbed by your skin.

- Even when you're driving your car you are exposed to the sun. If you are wearing a short-sleeve shirt, make sure you put sunscreen on your arms and hands.

- If you decide to wear a hat, it doesn't mean you should forego sunscreen. Apply it to your face and neck—and don't forget your ears, which can burn easily.

- The water is a tricky place. Not only do you risk having the sunscreen wash off your body, but the sun's reflection off the water increases the possibility of sunburn. Use waterproof sunblock and reapply after spending time in the water.

- If you live in a higher altitude you can burn more easily. Depending on your skin type, you may want to increase the level of the SPF you use.

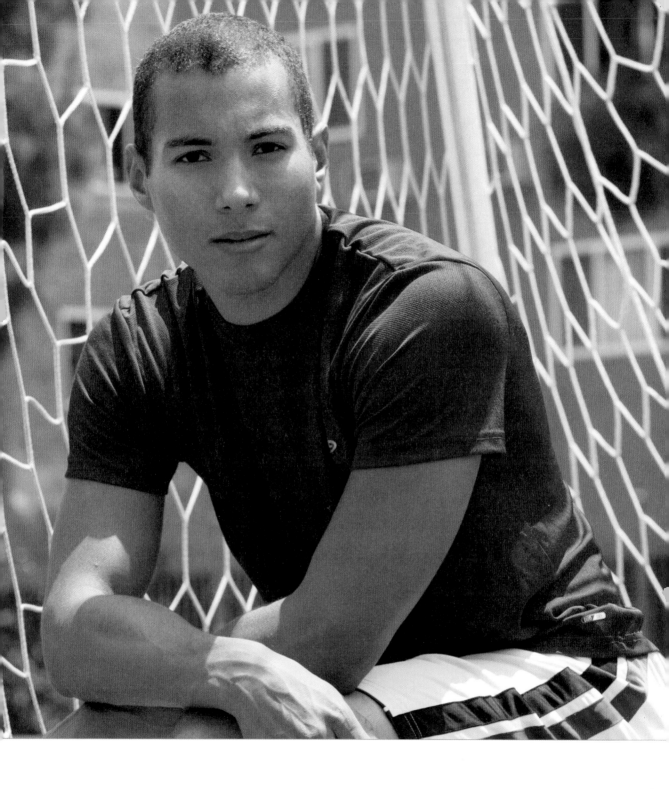

Men's Daily SPF Two-Step

Many men say it's hard to find a sunscreen that isn't too greasy. They find that the majority of the choices out there make them break out. This is especially the case during outdoor activities because men are sweating and many sunscreens clog pores. The goal is to select a brand that's not only good to the environment but also good to you.

Before heading outside, men should do two things: Apply an eco-friendly SPF cream that contains no titanium dioxide, petrochemicals, or artificial ingredients, and use an eco-friendly lip balm with SPF. The lips are sensitive and need to be protected, as well.

Here are my top picks for sun protection.

Alba Botanica Organic Lavender Sunscreen, SPF 30: Broad-spectrum UVA and UVB sun protection filled with 100 percent vegetarian ingredients and blended with certified organic herbs and antioxidants. It fights off the sun and fights off aging, as well. It's also pH balanced, good for all skin types, and hypoallergenic.

Eco Lips Organic Sport Lip Balm, SPF 30: This lip balm is made from vegetable oils, herbs, and beeswax, and it protects lips from harsh wind, cold, and sun.

I've Got Sunburn on a Cloudy Day

Even on a cloudy day, you can get a sunburn. If the clouds are light, as much as 80 percent of the sun's UV rays can make it through.

Surf's Up

It's very important to have on hand a sunscreen that is eco-friendly and water friendly. Living in California, I come into contact with a very large surfing community. Most surfers are not only loyal to the ocean, but also loyal to protecting it. When I began to research eco-friendly sunscreen options for men, I immediately asked my good friend Todd—a die-hard surfer and all around "green" guy—what the waterproof sunscreen of choice is among the surfing community. He raved about the virtues of Soléo Organics sunscreen.

Soléo Organics sunscreen (soleousa. com): This FDA-approved product is all natural and organically produced. It's free of UV absorbers, titanium dioxide, and synthetic preservatives. It's also biodegradable and has a low skin irritation factor.

MAN-i-Pedi

Nothing is more attractive to a woman than a well-groomed man from head to toe. Unkempt nails on your feet and hands, although tolerated, are not desired. Now, this doesn't mean your girlfriend or wife wants you to tag along on her weekly visit to the nail salon. Look to get a mani-pedi once a month. Keeping your fingernails and toenails groomed regularly is also good for your health because your nails carry germs that can transfer to other parts of your body. Furthermore, a mani-pedi is also a relaxing experience that can include a foot or hand massage. Don't forget to tip!

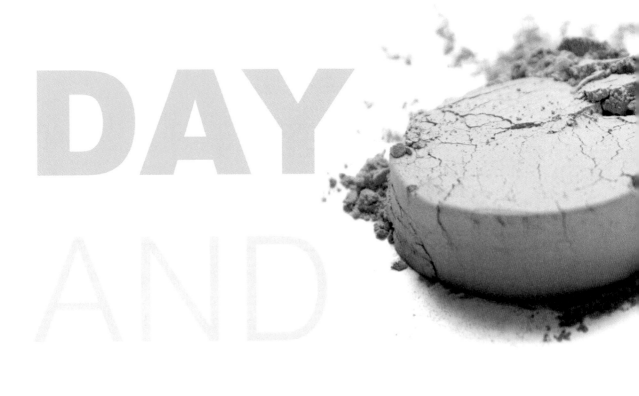

chapter 6

DAY AND NIGHT LOOKS

As children, all of us played "dress up." I remember getting glammed up with my friends, fixing each other's hair and putting on our mothers' makeup before our imaginary big night with Prince Charming. Today, creating different looks for women—transforming a client into whatever her heart desires—is one of my favorite parts of being a makeup artist. Whether it's a wedding, an awards show, or another significant event in a woman's life, I feel that I'm a part of their special day in some small way. It's fun, creative, and rewarding. When a client sees herself in the mirror and smiles, I know I've done my job.

When I first began to incorporate eco-friendly makeup into my sessions, many women would ask me if they could still get the sexy look they wanted by using "green" makeup. The answer is yes—and the proof is in these pages. Eco-friendly makeup feeds your skin nutrients while helping you achieve a sexy, sophisticated look. What could be better than that? It's all about understanding your skin type and using the products that work best for you.

Makeup application can create looks as dramatically different as night and day—literally. For a daytime look, you might want something professional yet sophisticated. An evening look could call for something a bit more sexy or glamorous for a night out on the town. It all depends on your specific needs: where you're going, what you're wearing, what kind of mood you're in. In this chapter, I am going to reveal some of my favorite looks for any daytime or nighttime occasion that comes your way.

SEIZE THE DAY

It's certainly true that a daytime look calls for something a bit more subtle than a nighttime look. However, that doesn't mean that it's any less important. Some of the most memorable experiences of our lives happen during the day. Whether it's a family barbecue, a baby shower, a wedding, or a board meeting at work, it's important to know how to create the appropriate look.

When it comes to creating a stunning daytime face, the key is to keep it simple yet sophisticated: Less is more. But just because you're using less makeup, that doesn't mean that your features can't still be flattered and brought to life.

By sharing my signature daytime looks—the No-Makeup Makeup Look, Business Chic, Fun and Flirty, and Bronzed Babe—I will show you how to combine and apply eco-friendly products that will help you achieve the perfect look for any daytime occasion. (See page 116.)

(Note: Before trying any of the following eco-beautiful daytime looks, follow the steps in Chapter 4 that describe how to apply the best foundation, concealer, and powder for your skin type.)

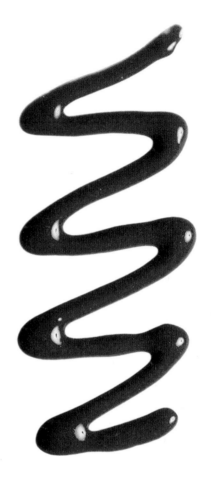

Workaday Beauty

Keep a few things tucked away in your office desk drawer to freshen up midday. I suggest always having a small mirror, blotting papers, hand cream, powder, lipstick, and/or lip gloss. This is all you need for a quick little touch-up that will help you look and feel refreshed.

The No-Makeup Makeup Look

The No-Makeup Makeup Look started a few years ago within the beauty and fashion industry. In all of the hottest fashion magazines, like *Vogue, Cosmo,* and *Glamour,* we began to see stunning, fresh-faced women who looked as if they weren't wearing any makeup…but they were! From glowing skin, to rosy cheeks, to supple lips, to the perfect brows, these gorgeous women were made up with a simple, subtle touch that highlighted their natural beauty. The idea of applying makeup to look as if you weren't wearing any makeup at all was a revelation to beauty industry insiders and consumers alike.

Even though the No-Makeup Makeup Look broke onto the scene a few years ago, it's still extremely popular. In fact, it's probably the most requested look in the industry. And I understand why. I believe that makeup's main role is to enhance a woman's beauty. This technique allows your natural beauty to shine through.

Here are my steps to achieving this look. It's simple and uncomplicated—and so is the application!

How to Apply

Apply a soft, gold, neutral shimmer shadow to your lids and gently brush it up to the crease. Take the same shimmer and apply it to the inner corner of the eye. It will brighten up the eye immediately. Smudge a brown eye pencil into your lash line. Remember to keep it as close to the lash line as possible. (This way it will look more natural.) Curl your lashes and apply a couple of coats of black mascara onto your upper and lower lashes. Apply a cream blush to the apples of your cheeks. (A cream blush will blend into your skin more easily and make your skin look like it's glowing from the inside out.) Lastly, the perfect finish to this look is a sheer pink or nude lip gloss. This will give your lips a pretty, natural shine.

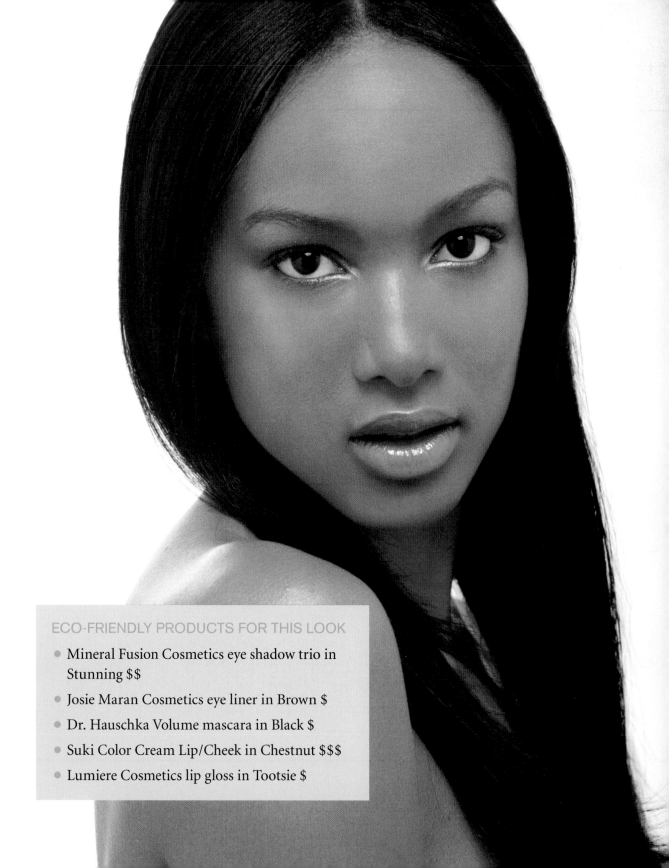

ECO-FRIENDLY PRODUCTS FOR THIS LOOK

- Mineral Fusion Cosmetics eye shadow trio in Stunning $$
- Josie Maran Cosmetics eye liner in Brown $
- Dr. Hauschka Volume mascara in Black $
- Suki Color Cream Lip/Cheek in Chestnut $$$
- Lumiere Cosmetics lip gloss in Tootsie $

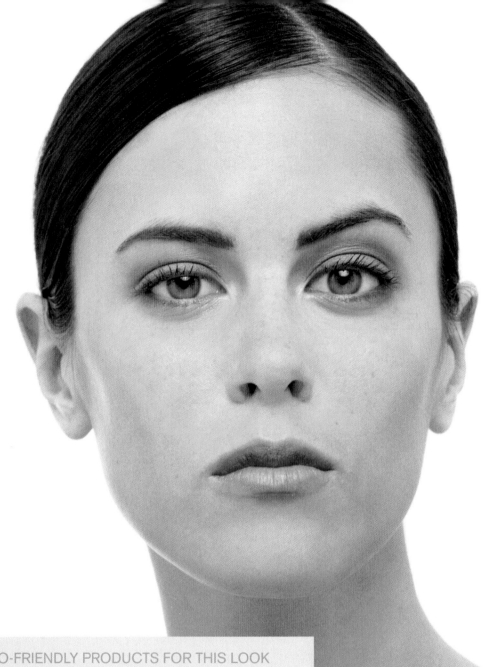

ECO-FRIENDLY PRODUCTS FOR THIS LOOK

- Mineral Fusion Cosmetics eye shadow trio in Fragile $$
- Bare Escentuals bareMinerals eye shadow in Java $
- Nvey Eco organic moisturizing mascara in Black $
- Mineral Fusion Cosmetics blush in Impact $
- Josie Maran Cosmetics lipstick in Flirtatious $

Business Chic

Beauty icon Marilyn Monroe once said "I don't mind living in a man's world as long as I can be a woman in it." Well, it's certainly not a man's world any longer, especially in the workplace. More than ever, women are thriving professionally as major business leaders. Whether you're already a CEO or are interviewing for your first job, one thing's for sure: You need to look polished and professional. The Business Chic look will get you noticed and help you command the respect and attention you deserve.

Believe it or not, your office may have more beauty obstacles than you think. For example, most corporate offices are lit by fluorescent bulbs, which can create very unflattering light. It may make you look pale and reveal imperfections in your skin that are less noticable in other light. And working long hours at the office eventually shows on our faces—tired eyes, smudged eye makeup, and dry lips. In this section, I'll teach you how to create my signature Business Chic look.

How to Apply

Apply a medium brown, taupy eye shadow to your lids and blend out well to the crease. Use the same shadow and smudge it out in your lower lashlines. Remember, no sharp lines. Wet a dark brown eye shadow and apply it as an eyeliner in your upper lash lines. Using a wet shadow as your eyeliner is a great trick—it gives you a more precise line, but doesn't look as harsh as an eyeliner. Next, take a white or nude eye pencil to the inside rims of your eyes. (This will open up the eye and make your eyes look more awake.) Then, sweep a couple of coats of black mascara onto your upper and lower lashes. Apply a rosy blush to the apples of your cheeks using a big blush brush. As for lips, choose a sheer rosy pink lip color in the same shade as your cheek color.

Fun and Flirty

During the day, you want to sport a look that's vibrant enough to get you noticed, but not to the point of distraction. Of course, we all have to let loose every once in a while and I am a strong believer that when appropriate, daytime makeup can be a little daring. Just use discretion—the corporate picnic is not the right time to glam it up. But, say you're invited to a weekend beach party—now *that's* the kind of event where you want to get your color on. And that's why I adore the Fun and Flirty look. It's an excuse to have some daytime fun!

Shades of turquoise, fuchsia, purple, and blue are all fabulous eye-color options for a Fun and Flirty daytime look. The trick with this look is not only to choose the right colors, but also to find the feature on your face that you want to enhance. You never want your eyes and lips to have to compete with each other. Here's how to achieve this fun look.

How to Apply

Use a brightly colored eyeliner to line your upper lashlines, lower lashlines, and the inside rims of your eyes. Repeat these steps two or three times to create a more dramatic look. Then curl your lashes and sweep a couple coats of a blue or purple mascara onto your upper and lower lashes. This will add extra color to your eyes and make them really pop. Choose a soft pink blush and apply it to the apples of your cheeks, to balance out the eye makeup. Leave your lips nude and apply a little lip balm to keep them moisturized throughout the day, especially if you're spending time outdoors.

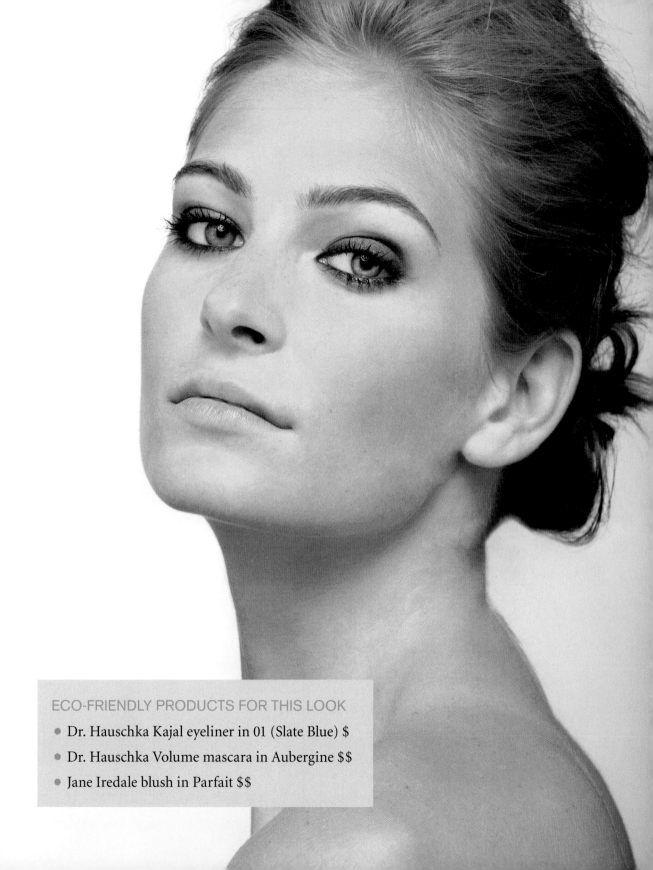

ECO-FRIENDLY PRODUCTS FOR THIS LOOK

- Dr. Hauschka Kajal eyeliner in 01 (Slate Blue) $
- Dr. Hauschka Volume mascara in Aubergine $$
- Jane Iredale blush in Parfait $$

Bronzed Babe

In Chapter 2 we discussed the dangers of the sun. According to many experts and studies, the sun is responsible for up to 95 percent of fine lines and wrinkles. That said, many women still love to sport a tan. At times, we all want that sultry bronzed glow that seems so simple and natural for women like Eva Mendes and Gisele Bündchen. So how do you get that gorgeous bronzed look without the sunshine? The answer: bronzer.

Using a quality eco-friendly bronzer is a fabulous way to achieve that healthy glow without damaging or aging your skin. The key to applying bronzer is to make sure it looks natural. You don't want your skin to look orange or streaky. In my Bronzed Babe look, I'll show you how to create your own supermodel-worthy glow.

How to Apply

Apply bronzer to the parts of your face where the sun would normally hit— forehead, cheeks, and nose. Apply a gold/bronze eye shadow to your eyelids and brush it up to the crease. Put the same color shadow on your brow bones to give your eyes a lift, and also on the inside corners of the eyes. Using a brown eye pencil, line the upper lash lines and the inside rims of the eyes. Curl your lashes and sweep two coats of black mascara onto your upper and lower lashes. Apply a shimmery, warm rose blush to the apples of your cheeks. Next, apply a gold shimmer to your temples. This will give your skin a truly glowing and beautiful look. Finish this look off by applying a pretty peach gloss with a hint of shimmer in it.

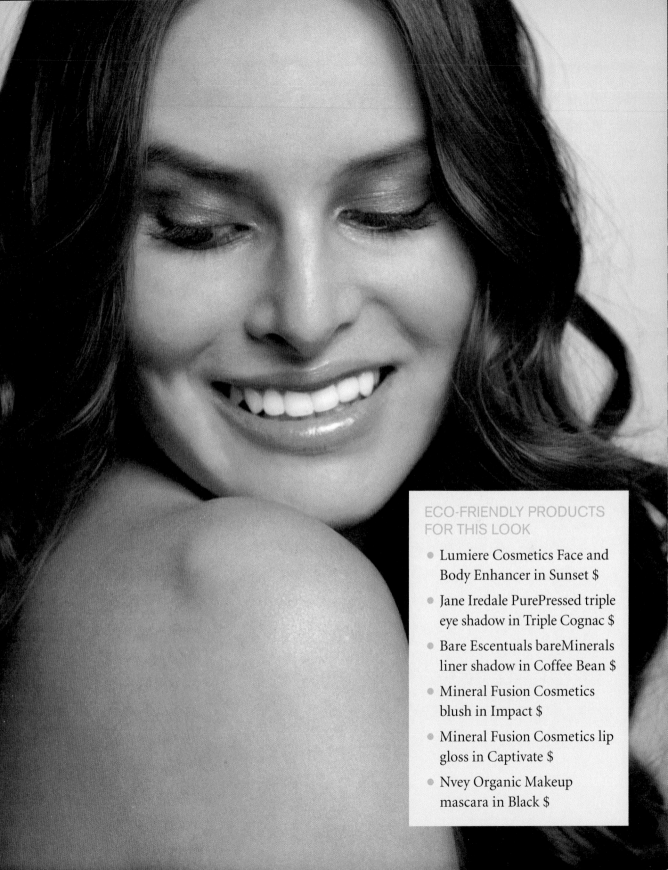

ECO-FRIENDLY PRODUCTS FOR THIS LOOK

- Lumiere Cosmetics Face and Body Enhancer in Sunset $
- Jane Iredale PurePressed triple eye shadow in Triple Cognac $
- Bare Escentuals bareMinerals liner shadow in Coffee Bean $
- Mineral Fusion Cosmetics blush in Impact $
- Mineral Fusion Cosmetics lip gloss in Captivate $
- Nvey Organic Makeup mascara in Black $

WHEN THE LIGHTS GO DOWN

Nighttime gives you the chance to try out a more daring makeup look. Whether you are headed out on a romantic dinner date or meeting up with the girls for cocktails on the town, you want to feel sexy and sophisticated. I love to create nighttime looks for my clients because I get the opportunity to really have fun and experiment. And the recipe for achieving this nighttime look is quite simple—create a little glam, add some drama, and you're definitely on your way to that makeup "wow factor" that will get you noticed!

With a nighttime look you can use different textures, shades, and colors. Don't be afraid to experiment and play around a little bit. You'll be surprised by the results. Just remember that any makeup look should have a focal point. For example, if you want to play up your eyes, opt for a neutral lip color, and vice versa. My four favorite nighttime looks focus on either the eyes or the lips: Metallic Maven, Green-Carpet Ready, Sexy Vixen, and Glamour Girl. I am going to show you how to get that irresistible, eco-friendly evening glow you've always wanted. When the lights go down, the fun begins, ladies!

(Note: Before trying any of the following eco-beautiful nighttime looks, follow the steps in Chapter 4 that describe how to apply the best foundation, concealer, and powder for your skin type.)

Lip Tip
Drink beverages from a straw to avoid messing up your lip gloss or lipstick.

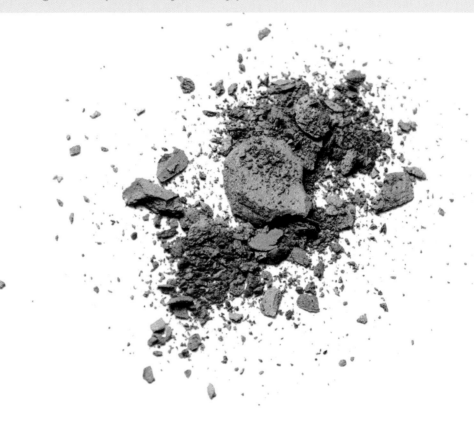

Metallic Maven

Metallics can create an eye-catching look and are a great way to add a bit of spark and excitement to your face. Trendy shades like silver, metallic blue, gold, and bronze can really make for a winning evening makeup look. Metallics add that "fun factor" when you're getting glammed up for an exciting night out on the town. In fact, Metallic

Maven is a fabulous look to wear to a nightclub.

In my experience, metallics work their magic best when they're worn on either your eyelids or your lips. It's all about deciding which will be your focal point. Also, be sure not to layer the metallic look: Just one layer of metallic eye shadow or cream shadow will go a long way. Follow the steps below and you will become a Metallic Maven in no time!

How to Apply

If your eyes are the focal point, apply a metallic shade of your choice to your eyelids. Gently brush the shadow up to the crease. Take the same metallic shade and apply it to your lower lash lines as well as to the inside corners of your eyes. This will make your eyes pop. Then, choose a lighter metallic shade in the same color family. (For example, if you are working with a bronze shade, use a gold shimmer. If you are working with navy or gray metallics, choose a

silver or frosty white shade.) Apply this to the inside corners of the eyes and in the center of the eyelids. This will create a gorgeous 3-D look. Using an eye pencil in gray or brown (depending on the metallic shades you are using), line the inside rims of your eyes. This will give a more dramatic feel to your look. Curl your lashes, and sweep a couple of coats of black mascara onto your upper and lower lashes. If you want, apply a subtle cream blush to your cheeks, using your fingers. You want to keep the cheeks as subtle as possible because you want the eyes to be the focal point. Lastly, sweep a nice, nude brown gloss over your lips for the perfect final touch to this nighttime look.

If you'd prefer for your lips to be the focal point, opt for a darker, richer shade of lipstick, like a wine or burgundy that contains a hint of shimmer. Keep the rest of your makeup subtle by applying a lighter eyeshadow to your lids and a couple of coats of black or brown mascara.

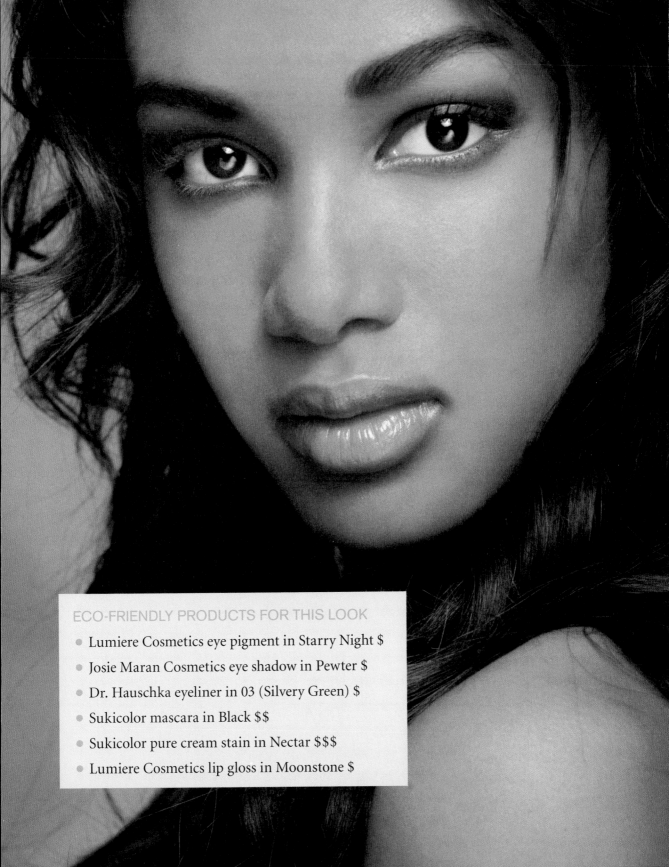

ECO-FRIENDLY PRODUCTS FOR THIS LOOK

- Lumiere Cosmetics eye pigment in Starry Night $
- Josie Maran Cosmetics eye shadow in Pewter $
- Dr. Hauschka eyeliner in 03 (Silvery Green) $
- Sukicolor mascara in Black $$
- Sukicolor pure cream stain in Nectar $$$
- Lumiere Cosmetics lip gloss in Moonstone $

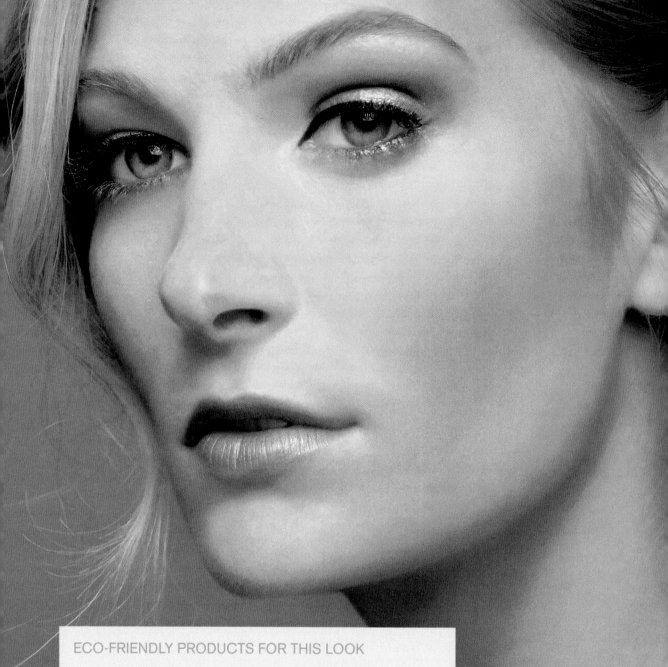

ECO-FRIENDLY PRODUCTS FOR THIS LOOK

- Lumiere Cosmetics eye pigment in Hypnotic $
- Ecco Bella soft eyeliner pencil in Velvet $
- Ecco Bella FlowerColor natural mascara in Black $
- Lumiere Cosmetics face and body enhancer in Starstruck $
- Josie Maran Cosmetics lipstick in Curvaceous $

Green-Carpet Ready

I've created red-carpet looks for a variety of celebrities for events such as the Academy Awards, the Golden Globes, and the Grammy Awards. I love having the opportunity to help an actor get ready for her big night. These days, it seems there are just as many green-carpet events as red-carpet events. Environmental award ceremonies such as the Green Cross Awards and the Green House Project roll out the green carpet instead of a red one when they host events, to bring further awareness to their important environmental causes.

Whether I do a woman's makeup for a red- or green-carpet event, I like to add a little something extra. After all, their pictures will appear in countless magazines—their makeup really has to dazzle. But you don't have to be a celebrity to get a green-carpet look. Maybe you have an invitation to a fancy dinner party, a holiday party, a wedding, or a charity gala. You need a special makeup look for your special occasion. Wherever you are headed, this will make you look like a star!

How to Apply

First, choose an eye color that has a little sparkle. Try a shade of green, navy, plum, or terra-cotta. Apply the color to your eyelids and blend up to the crease. Next, apply a dark brown or black eye pencil to the inside rims of your eyes. Curl your lashes and glue on false eyelash strips to the lashes. Let them dry for a few minutes, and sweep some black mascara onto your upper and lower lashes. Apply a shimmery blush to the apples of your cheeks. Last, apply a darker pink lipstick to your lips with a lip brush, which will help you apply with more precision.

Sexy Vixen

Combine a little attitude with a smoky eye, and you're on your way to becoming a Sexy Vixen! A smoky eye is chic and sexy and will boost your confidence in seconds.

The really fun thing about a smoky eye is that you don't have to go with a traditional black shade. The way to achieve an ultra-fabulous smoky eye is to pick a shade that works for your skin tone. If you have fair skin, a black smoky eye can look too dramatic. Instead, pick shades of brown. Additionally, plums, moss greens, browns, and grays can also create a beautiful smoky eye. Remember, nighttime looks are about being daring, and a smoky eye *is* daring!

(Note: For more information about choosing the correct eye shadow shade for your eye color, turn to Chapter 4.)

How to Apply

Using a dark-colored eye pencil of your choice, line your upper and lower lash lines as well as the inside rims of your eyes. (If you are doing a brown smoky eye, choose a dark brown eye pencil; if you are doing a black smoky eye, choose a black eye pencil.) Smudge out the lines with a cotton swab or your fingertip. Apply the dark eye shadow to your eyelids and blend it out well to the crease using an eco-friendly eye shadow brush. Go over this step a couple of times to intensify the effect. Apply the same eye shadow using a slightly thinner eye shadow brush under your lower lash lines. Make sure to smudge it out well. No sharp lines! Take a white shimmer cream or powder shadow and apply it on your brow bones and on the inside corners of your eyes. This will add some depth to your eyes and make your eye makeup look more complete. Curl your lashes and sweep two coats of black mascara onto your upper and lower lashes. Apply a soft pink cream or powder blush to the apples of your cheeks. This will make your blush look like a healthy and natural flush. Lastly, apply a nude lipstick or a gloss.

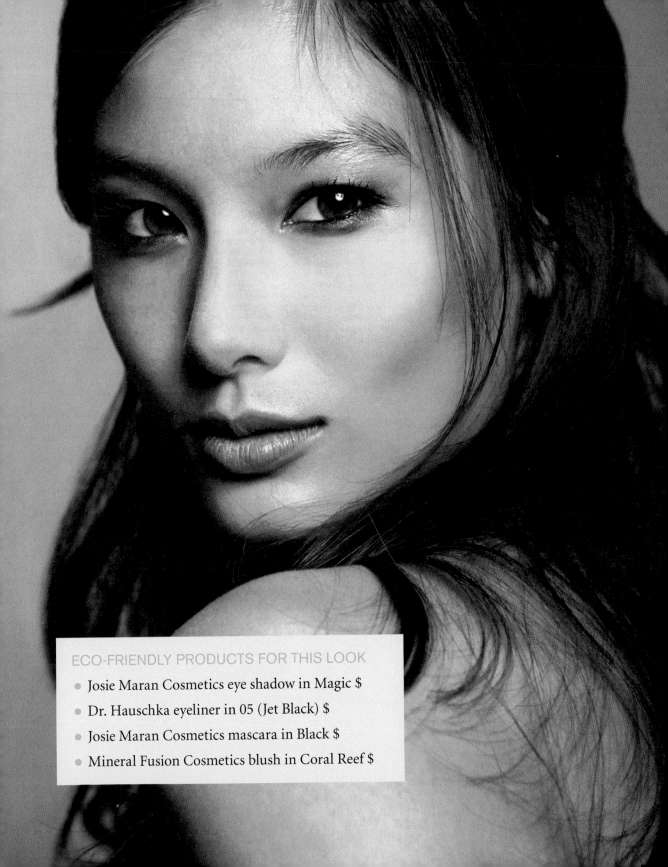

ECO-FRIENDLY PRODUCTS FOR THIS LOOK

- Josie Maran Cosmetics eye shadow in Magic $
- Dr. Hauschka eyeliner in 05 (Jet Black) $
- Josie Maran Cosmetics mascara in Black $
- Mineral Fusion Cosmetics blush in Coral Reef $

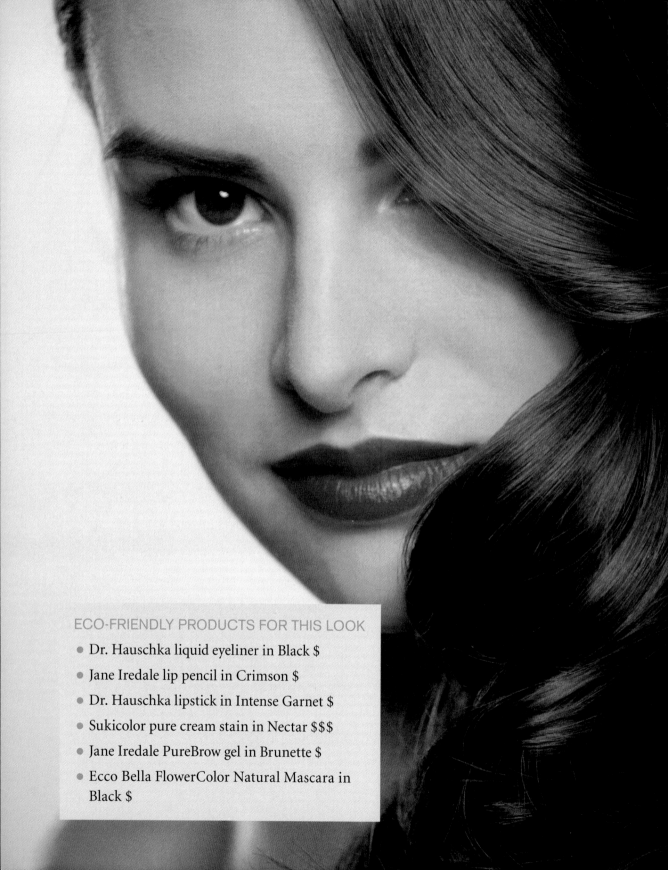

ECO-FRIENDLY PRODUCTS FOR THIS LOOK

- Dr. Hauschka liquid eyeliner in Black $
- Jane Iredale lip pencil in Crimson $
- Dr. Hauschka lipstick in Intense Garnet $
- Sukicolor pure cream stain in Nectar $$$
- Jane Iredale PureBrow gel in Brunette $
- Ecco Bella FlowerColor Natural Mascara in Black $

Glamour Girl

We all want to look extra glamorous sometimes, and I believe a sultry red lip truly exudes glamour! Glamour Girl is a classic look that will never go out of style. Think Veronica Lake and old Hollywood: long, slinky gowns; platform shoes; luxurious, wavy hair; and a bold red lip. A lot of women seem to be afraid of red lipstick. In my experience, their fear stems from the idea that it is difficult to find a shade of red that complements their skin tone. But I assure you, it's not hard to figure out.

All women basically fall into two skin-tone categories: cool tones and warm tones. To find the best red lip shade for you, follow the steps below. Once you've chosen your lip color, you can begin the makeup application and go out and paint the town red . . . literally!

Cool tones. If your skin has pink undertones (generally blondes with pale skin), choose red lip shades like berry reds and brick reds.

Warm tones. If your skin has more of a yellow undertone (generally with brunettes and darker skin), choose red lip shades like orangey reds, tomato reds, and brown reds.

How to Apply

Sweep a black liquid eyeliner as close to your upper lash lines as possible. This will make your lashes look thicker and fuller. Then, drag the liner out and up at the outer ends of your lash lines to create "wings." This eye makeup works perfectly with red lips; It looks classy and elegant. Curl your lashes and apply two coats of black mascara to your upper and lower lashes. Next, sweep a tinted brow gel gently across the arch of your brows to help define them and add a hint of color. Then apply a cream blush or stain on the apples of your cheeks, using your fingers. Before you apply the lipstick to help define your lips, shade the entire lip area using a lip liner. This will make your lipstick last longer, so you won't have to reapply as often. Lastly, apply a sultry red lipstick using a lip brush.

chapter 7

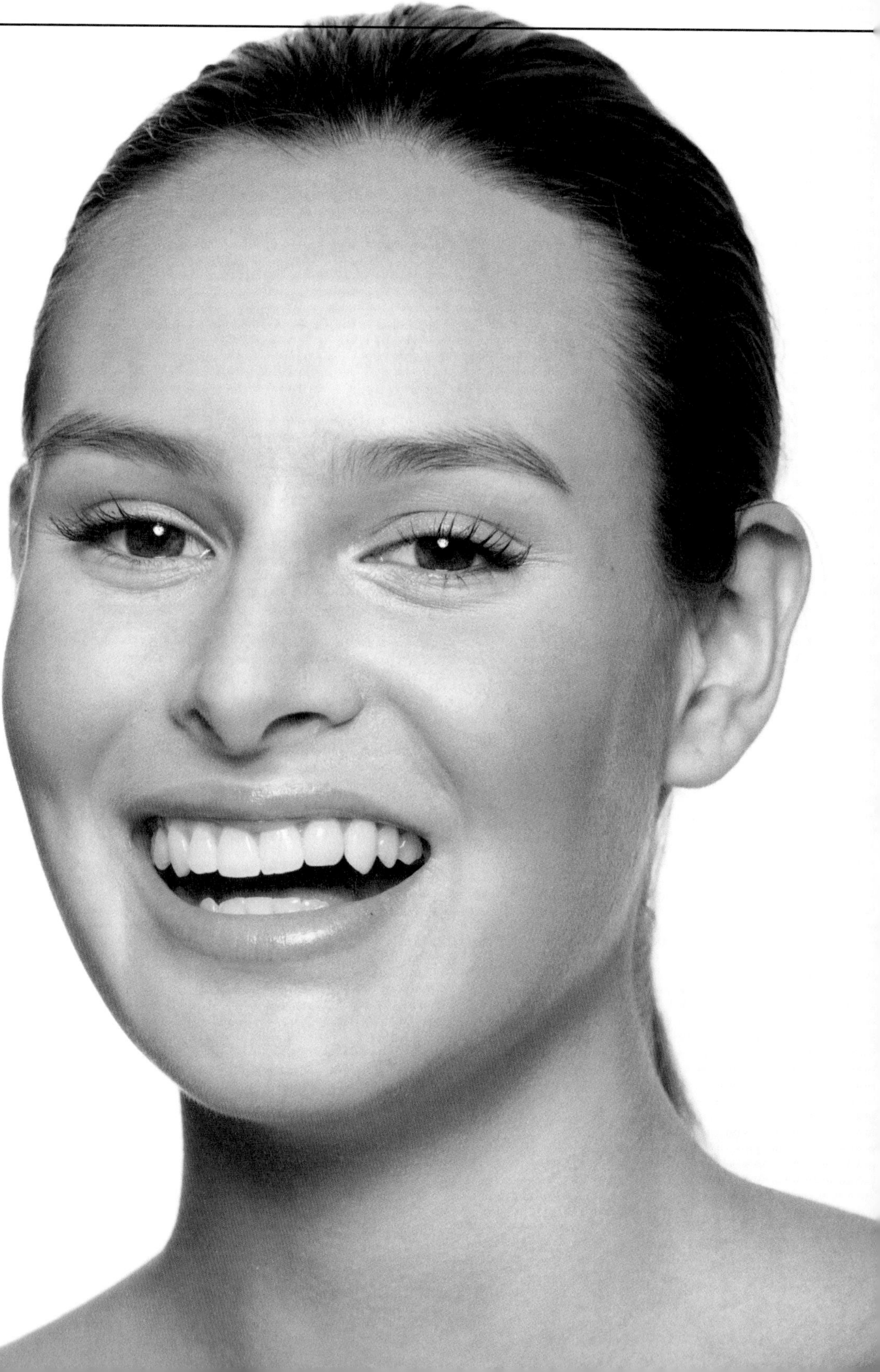

TIMELESS ECO-BEAUTY

As a makeup artist, it's exciting to work with cutting-edge trends. But I also enjoy creating timeless looks. When I think of classic beauty, I think of icons like Marilyn Monroe and Audrey Hepburn. Their looks were one-of-a-kind, and their beauty truly defined the word timeless. The styles these ladies inspired can be just as fresh and fun as the latest trends.

In this chapter, I'll introduce you to some classic, fun, and chic looks that are sure to work for any season, lifestyle, or age. I guarantee you will find a look that will suit your needs and hopefully ignite some creative new ideas.

I will offer you seasonal colors that inspire me and make me feel alive. For instance, during the spring months, I love working with colors like peach, apricot, and pink. They generate the spirit of freshness associated with that time of the year. I will also introduce you to various women from all walks of life whose age-appropriate makeup looks will reflect style and sophistication, while highlighting their best features.

Eco-friendly makeup is the present and future of cosmetics—so let's get started on some timeless looks . . .

THE FOUR SEASONS

If there's one thing that I truly miss living in Los Angeles, it's the four seasons. When I was growing up in Sweden and when I lived in London and New York City, I looked forward to the seasonal weather changes, especially during the spring and fall months. There's nothing like the first crisp, cool, fall day after a long, hot summer. Or the sight of a crystal blue spring sky after a dark, frigid winter.

Regardless of where we live, we all have to adapt our beauty regimen for each season. Changes in the weather and temperature can take a serious toll on our skin. We need to protect ourselves from whatever Mother Nature decides to throw our way. For instance, during the summer heat, our skin is more prone to breakouts. I recommend using mineral makeup during the hot, humid months of July and August. Mineral makeup allows the skin to breathe and helps to neutralize the oils on the skin. During the winter months, I recommend using a liquid or cream foundation, which will help keep the skin moisturized.

In this chapter I detail each of my

favorite eco-beautiful looks for the four seasons. Remember that each season gives you an opportunity to try something different and exciting. When fall hits, you should go for a more earthy style by using shades of green, brown, and plum. In winter, colors like navy and black are your ticket to a more dramatic and sultry appearance. For spring, you want to sport a look that's simple, fresh, and pretty. During the summer, I suggest opting for bright colors and pastels. This section is all about getting you "green" and glamorous all year round!

Fabulous Colors for the Four Seasons

Fall	Winter	Spring	Summer
Plum	Silver	Peach	Turquoise
Wine	Red	Apricot	Lavender
Brown	Navy	Cream	Rose
Gold	Black	Beige	Bronze
Moss Green	Gray	Pink	Baby Blue

(Note: Before trying any of the following seasonal eco-beautiful looks, follow the steps in Chapter 4 that describe how to apply the best foundation, concealer, and powder for your skin type.)

The Order of Things

I use heavy eye makeup in some of the seasonal looks in this chapter. When creating a dramatic eye, a good trick is to apply it *before* you apply the foundation and concealer. Why? Sometimes the powder from the shadows can fall down on your face and smudge or mess up your foundation. Save yourself the trouble of reapplying by making foundation your last step.

Awww-tumn (fall look)

How to Apply

Apply a moss green shadow to your lids and gently brush it up to the crease. Make sure there are no sharp edges. Take the same moss green color and apply it in your lower lash lines and smudge it out. Next, layer a brown bronzy shadow over the green shadow using a bigger, fluffy brush. Use a brown eye pencil to line the inside rims of your eyes. Then, curl your lashes and apply a couple of coats of black mascara. Next, take an apricot-colored blush and apply it to the apples of your cheeks. This will instantly warm up your face and give it an autumn glow. Lastly, apply a wine-colored lipstick, using a lip brush to get a more precise application, to balance out this eco-beautiful makeup look.

ECO-FRIENDLY PRODUCTS FOR THIS LOOK

- Jane Iredale eye shadow trio in Khaki Craze $$
- Lumiere Cosmetics eye pigment in Soft Brown $
- Josie Maran Cosmetics eye liner in Brown $
- Jane Iredale PurePressed blush in Golden Apricot $$
- Josie Maran Cosmetics lipstick in Adventurous $
- Sukicolor Rich Pigment mascara in Black Velvet $$

Fall Tip

The first thing I do when I feel the chill of autumn is switch my daily moisturizer. Your skin tends to get a bit drier in the fall and winter, so opt for an eco-friendly cream that is heavier than what you would use in the summer months.

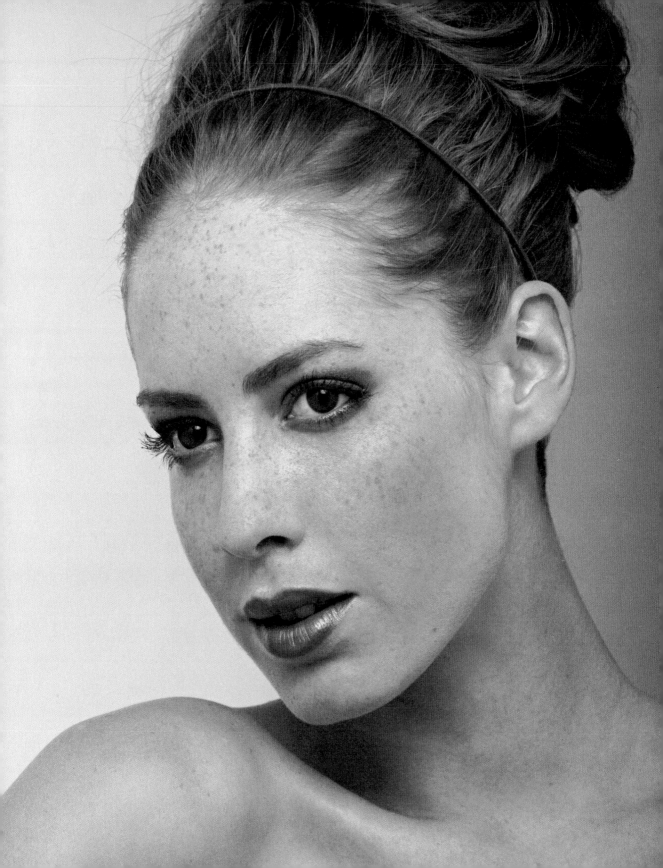

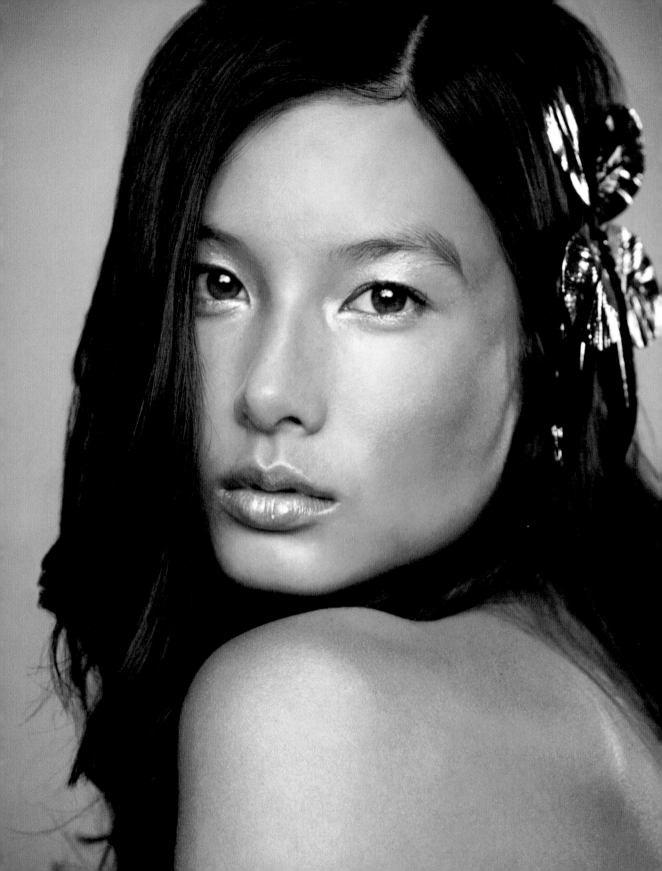

Cool Chick (winter look)

How to Apply

Apply a white or cream-colored shimmer shadow on your eyelids and brush it up to your brow bones. Take the same color shimmer and apply it on the inner corners of your eyes, right in the lower lash lines. Take a white eye pencil and apply it to the inside rims of your eyes. Curl your lashes and apply one coat of black mascara. Next, take a light pink blush with a touch of shimmer and apply it right on your cheekbones. The focus of this look is to keep everything very light and cool with frosty, shimmery shades. Apply a light, frosty, shimmer lip gloss to your lips for the perfect finish.

ECO-FRIENDLY PRODUCTS FOR THIS LOOK

- Lumiere Cosmetics Ditto eye color in 02 $$
- Jane Iredale eye highlighter pencil $
- Bare Escentuals bareMinerals cheek color in Sorbet $
- Josie Maran Cosmetics lip gloss in Radiance $
- Josie Maran Cosmetics mascara in Black $

Winter Tip

During the cold winter months, your hands are the first to suffer from dryness and cracking. Moisturize your hands and feet with a shea butter-based lotion before putting on gloves and socks in the morning and again before bedtime.

Spring Fling (spring look)
How to Apply

Apply a lavender or pink shimmery shadow on your eyelids and then brush it all the way up to your brow bones. Take a white shimmer shadow and apply it on the inside corners of your eyes. Next, take a dark brown eye pencil and use it as a liner right on your upper lash lines. Curl your lashes and apply two coats of black mascara. For the cheeks, opt for a light pink blush with a touch of shimmer in it. Lastly, choose a light pink pastel lipstick, and apply it with a lip brush.

ECO-FRIENDLY PRODUCTS FOR THIS LOOK

- Jane Iredale PurePressed triple eye shadow in Think Pink $
- Mineral Fusion Cosmetics eye pencil in Rough $
- Dr. Hauschka Volume mascara in Black $
- Mineral Fusion Cosmetics blush in Trace $
- Mineral Fusion Cosmetics lipstick in Impressive $

Spring Tip

After the cold winter months, take a moment in April to rub a mixture of honey and salt all over your body to moisturize and exfoliate. It eliminates dead skin cells, while leaving a smooth finish. After this, you can finally wear that skirt you been thinking about all winter long!

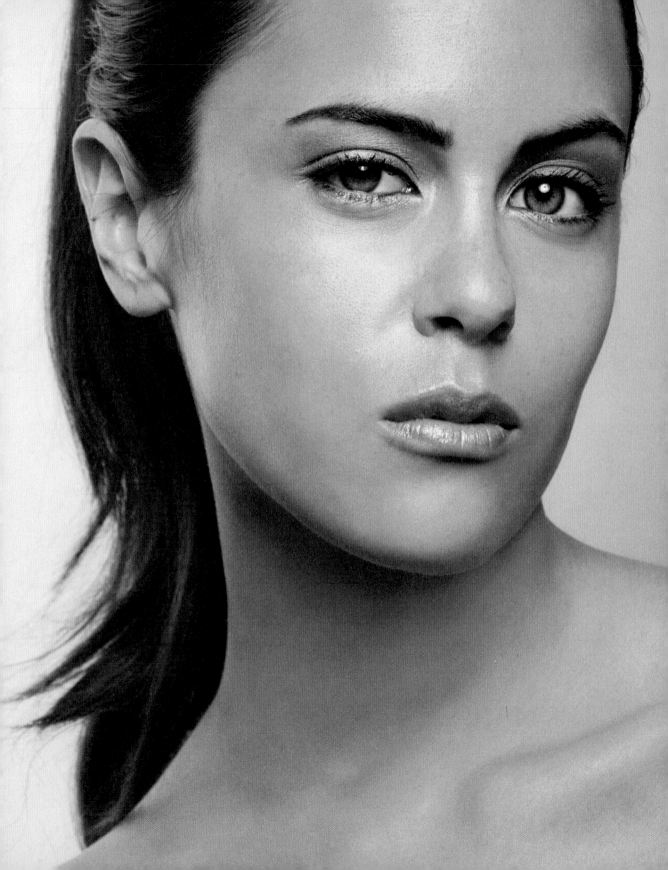

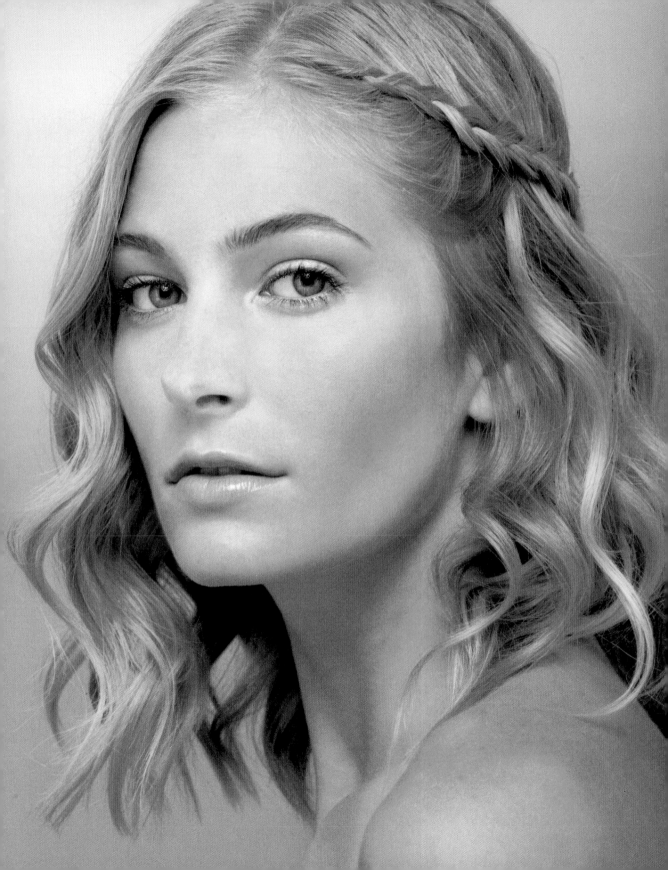

Hot Stuff (summer look)

How to Apply

Apply a gold shimmer shadow to your eyelids. Apply the same color on the inside corners of your eyes. Next, take a soft brown shadow and apply it on the crease, blending it out well. Next, take a white eye pencil and line the inside rims of your eyes. (This will open up the eye.) Curl your eyelashes and apply two coats of brown mascara, which will create less definition in the eye and will give you a softer eye look. Add a warm peach blush to the apples of your cheeks. Lastly, add a touch of peach-colored lip gloss.

ECO-FRIENDLY PRODUCTS FOR THIS LOOK

- Josie Maran Cosmetics eye shadow in Fairytale $
- Josie Maran Cosmetics eye shadow in Oak $
- Jane Iredale eye pencil in White $
- Dr. Hauschka mascara in Brown $$
- Dr. Hauschka rouge powder in 02 $$
- Jane Iredale PureGloss in Apricot Fizz $

Summer Tip

When the summer hits, I love bringing color back into my life. You will be baring your feet over these months, so take a look in the latest fashion magazines and find the nail polish colors of the season. Pick an eco-friendly polish that will be fun in the sun! (See page 89 for suggestions.)

BEAUTY FOR ALL AGES

We all know that things change as we age. And when it comes to your skin, you will undoubtedly notice change through the years. While makeup can always be used to enhance your appearance, it's important to create a look that suits your age, your personal style, and your life. What looks great on a woman in her twenties may not be quite as flattering on someone in her forties. It's also important to consider your daily beauty needs. A single woman with an active social life has a different set of priorities and beauty goals than a woman who is married and has children. It's all about where you are in your life at the moment.

Throughout the following pages, I'll introduce you to women from all walks of life who vary in age from their twenties to their fifties. And while each of these women is different, they all share a common desire to learn more about their own skin and how they can be more conscious of the environment.

I sat down with each woman to find out more about her specific skin issues and cosmetics goals. They each shared their beauty stories with me, and now I'll share them with you.

NAME: *Coco Knudson*

When I was younger, my mother owned a clothing store. She used to put on amazing fashion shows and my favorite part was to watch all the models get made up in extravagant makeup and hair. I first learned about makeup from my mom and she has been a great teacher.

Age: 19

Occupation: Student

Ethnicity: Caucasian

Skin type: Combination

Relationship status: In a relationship

I currently lead a standard college lifestyle. I'm trying to balance academics with extracurricular activities. I never have enough time to get ready in the mornings. With combination skin, I constantly battle occasional breakouts. But, with consistent care, my skin stays fairly normal. As I have gotten older my breakouts have become much more manageable and my skin has become a bit dryer.

I would love to learn some techniques for better makeup application and find out how I can adjust my look for day and night.

How to Apply

Experimenting with fun colors is the best part of being young. Keep this look light and fun using pastels. Start out by applying a light pastel color (in this case, a turquoise shadow) to your eyelids and all the way up to your brow bones. You still want to keep the colors light, so the look works well for both day and evening. Next, take a dark brown or black eye pencil and line your upper lash lines. Stay as close to the lash line as possible and smudge out using your fingertips. Curl your lashes and apply two coats of black mascara. For your cheeks, opt for a light pink blush to brighten up your face. Apply it on the apples of your cheeks using an eco-friendly blush brush. Finish off the look by applying a coat of a light pink shimmer lip gloss.

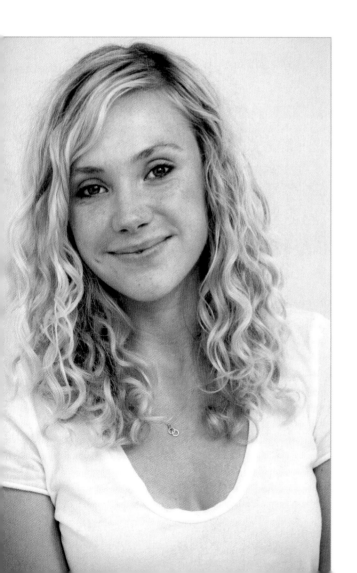

ECO-FRIENDLY PRODUCTS FOR THIS LOOK

- Nvey Eco organic eye shadow in Turquoise Shimmer $
- Mineral Fusion Cosmetics eye pencil in Coal $
- Ecco Bella FlowerColor natural mascara in Black $
- Bare Escentuals bareMinerals blush in Kiss $
- Dr. Hauschka Novum lip gloss in Rose Quartz $

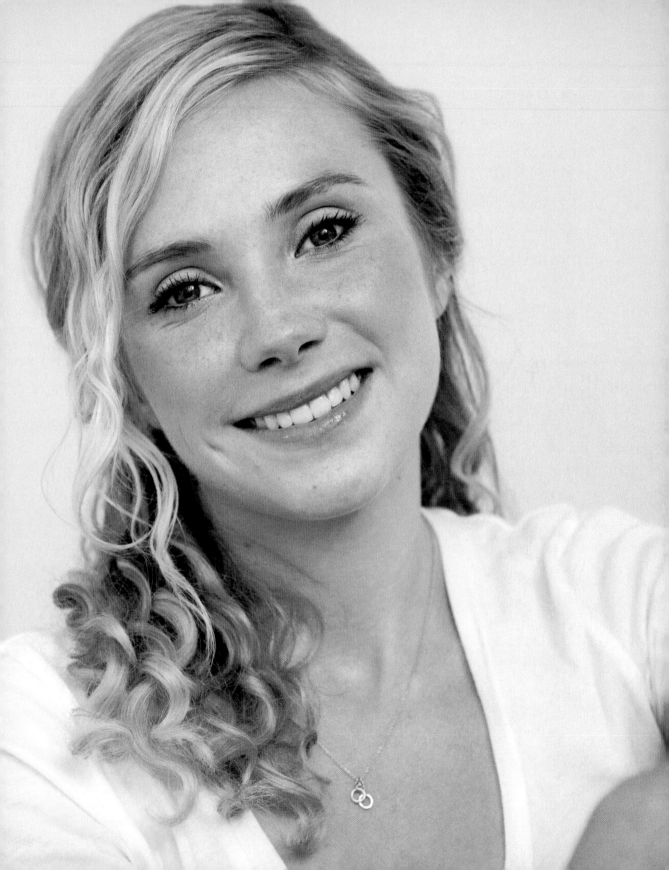

NAME: *Genevieve Cortese*

Age: 27

Occupation: Actress

Ethnicity: Caucasian
(Italian, Flemish, and German)

Skin type: Combination

Relationship status: Single

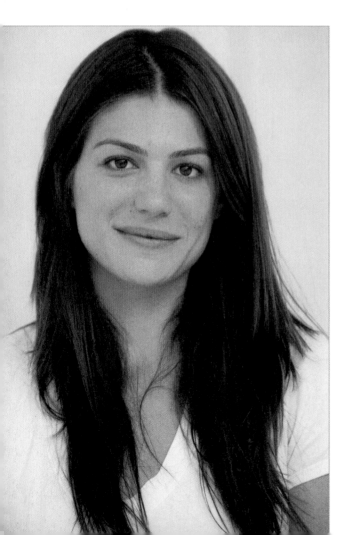

My mom hardly ever wore much makeup, which is probably why I don't wear a lot of it myself. In fact, I don't think that I started wearing makeup until I was in college. However, now that I'm a "grown-up," I've found that I've become much more feminine and a definite part of being a woman is dressing up. I probably spend around 10 minutes at most doing my makeup.

When I'm not working, I'm on the go a lot and live a pretty active lifestyle, so I try to stick to makeup looks that are quick and easy. My goals are pretty basic. As long as it's low maintenance, I'm in! One of my focuses is to be more "green." I would like a look that will afford me time, looks pretty, and is good to the environment.

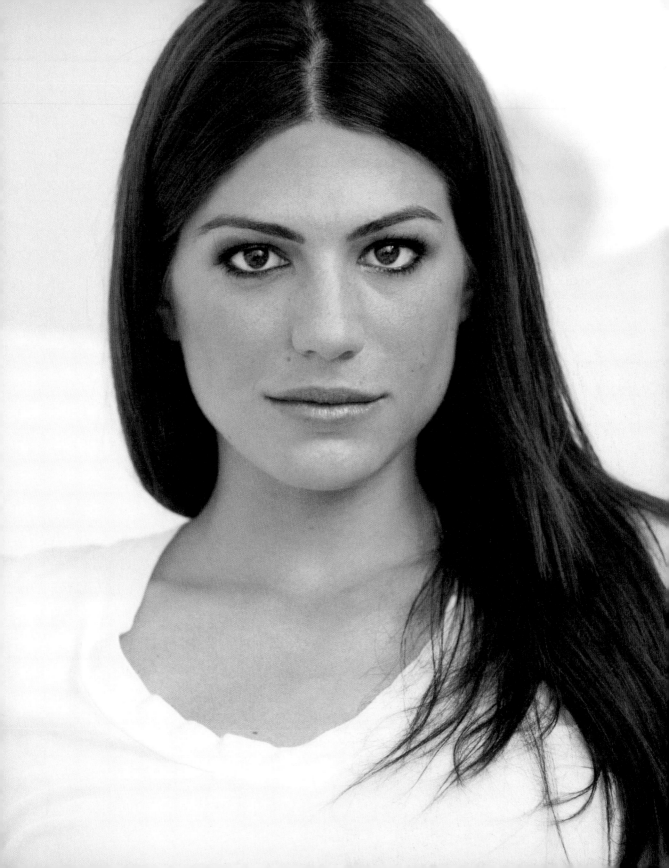

How to Apply

Most twentysomethings live a pretty hectic lifestyle. They also tend to want to experiment with makeup a bit more. Whether it's a day at work or a night out on the town, it's the perfect time to try something different using new colors. Choose one focal point. In this case, we decided to play up Genevieve's gorgeous brown eyes. To make this look your own, start out by applying a dark plum shadow to your eyelids and gently brush it up to the crease. Apply the same shadow to your lower lash lines and smudge out using your fingertips. You may have to repeat this to get the desired shade you want. Next, take a dark gray eye pencil and create a line as close to your upper lash lines as possible. Using the same pencil, line the inside rims of your eyes. To create a more dramatic look, apply a lighter plum shimmer right on the center of your eyelids. (This will also add more depth to the eye.) Curl your eyelashes and apply a couple of coats of black mascara. Next, sweep a soft pink blush on the apples of your cheeks. Keep the blush light, so it doesn't compete with the heavier eye look. Lastly, apply a coat of pink lip gloss to complete the look.

ECO-FRIENDLY PRODUCTS FOR THIS LOOK

- Jane Iredale PurePressed eye shadow triple in Cloud Nine $
- Mineral Fusion Cosmetics eye pencil in Volcanic $
- Josie Maran Cosmetics mascara in Black $
- Lumiere Cosmetics blush in Spiced Apple $
- Mineral Fusion Cosmetics lip gloss in Dazzle $

NAME: *Ansu Singh*

I first started using makeup when I was attending university. I got more into makeup after gradua- tion, when I began working full- time in the business world. I dressed in a business suit every day and found makeup to be an important part of my appearance.

Age: 33

Occupation: Sharebroker; temporarily taking a time-out as a ski bum

Ethnicity: Indian

Skin type: Normal

Relationship status: Single

A few years ago, I left the corporate world to travel. Traveling has certainly affected my skin a lot. Sometimes the change in my skin can be quite dra- matic, especially in relation to hydration or the lack thereof.

I plan on heading back to the corpo- rate world in the near future. I'm looking forward to learning how to create a classic makeup look that can go from wearing a business suit during the day all the way through to the evening, for a night out on the town after work.

How to Apply

If you're in your thirties, you prob- ably live a busy lifestyle and you need a look that might work for both day and night. I decided to use colors like brown and gold, which are great for daytime but also work for nighttime. Start out by applying a brown shadow to your eyelids. Blend well and brush up to the crease. Take a slightly lighter brown shadow and apply it right in your lower lash lines. Next, take a gold shimmer shadow and apply it on the inside corners of your eyes as well as on your eyelids. Curl your lashes and apply two coats of black mascara to your upper and lower lashes. Next, sweep a warm peach-colored blush on the apples of your cheeks. This will tie in nicely with the warm tones of the eye makeup. Apply a coat of lip gloss in a peachy shade.

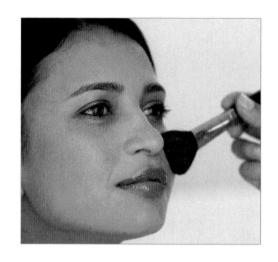

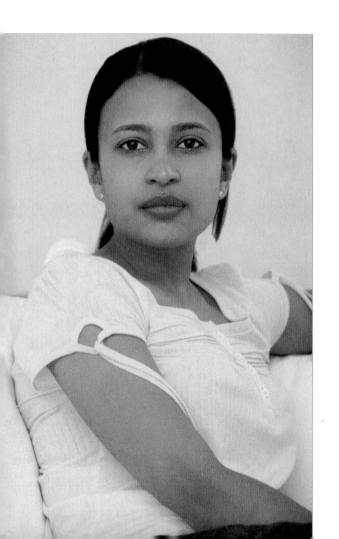

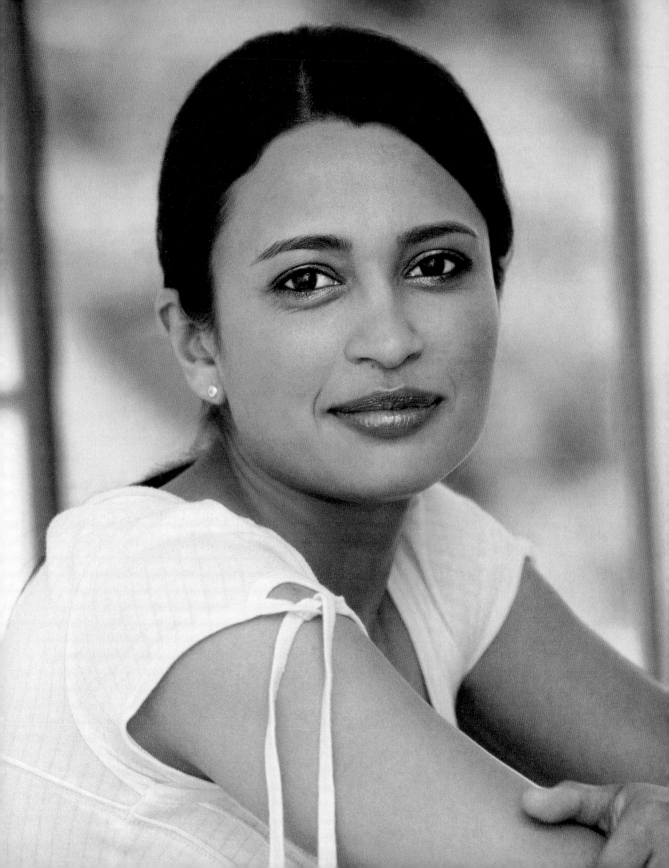

NAME: *Anne Litt*

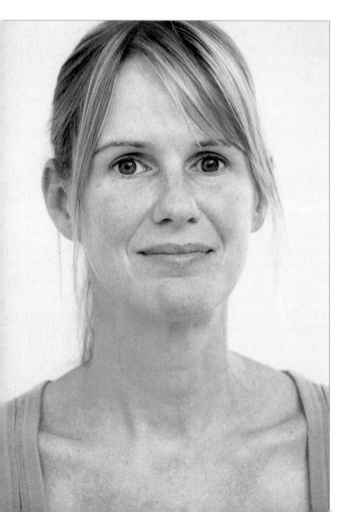

Age: 42

Occupation: DJ/Music supervisor/Mom

Ethnicity: Caucasian (English and Scottish)

Skin type: Mostly dry

Relationship status: Married with 2-year-old son

I was first introduced to makeup by my best friend's mom in the 1970s. She wore robin's egg blue eye shadow, and I thought she was so cool. My friend Beth and I would spend hours applying all the makeup (eye shadow in particular) that we could find.

My skin has gotten drier over the years. As I've grown older, rosacea has become more of a problem. It's important for me to look professional and put together. It's harder to get away with the casual college girl thing now that I'm in my forties. Having a baby has also really changed my feelings about needing and wanting to look good. When your body and lifestyle changes so much, it becomes important to keep your looks together.

As the mother of a 2-year-old, I rarely wear makeup during the day. I usually save it for going out at night.

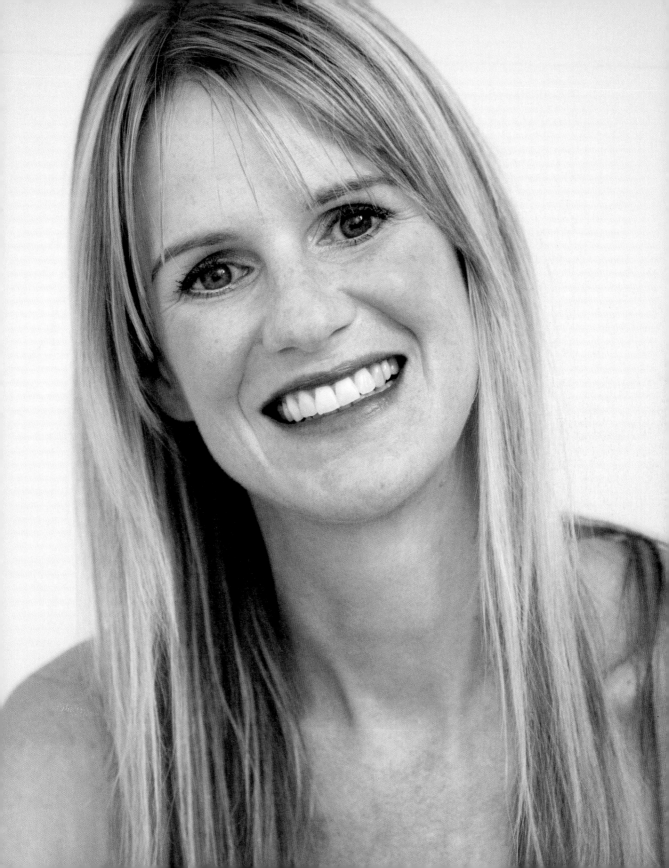

I would like to have a simple eco-friendly makeup routine that I could follow quickly in the morning, because I do feel like I need it.

How to Apply

In your forties, you may not have the same amount of time to spend on your makeup application as you did in your twenties. Being a mother and working a full-time job, you may not have more than 10 minutes to do your makeup in the morning. Creating a quick and easy makeup look that will brighten your face and last long is key! Start out by applying a lighter beige color to your eyelid. This will instantly brighten up any eye. Next, take a medium brown shadow and apply it right on the crease. Use the same color and apply it right in your lower lash lines. This will open up the eyes. Blend well. Next, use a dark brown eye pencil and line your upper lash lines. Curl your lashes and apply two coats of black mascara to the upper and lower lashes. Next, sweep a warm-colored blush on the apples of your cheeks and finish off this look by applying a warm terra-cotta shade of lipstick using a lip brush. This is a quick and simple makeup look that will make you look awake and healthy!

ECO-FRIENDLY PRODUCTS FOR THIS LOOK
- Lumiere Cosmetics eye pigment in Rested $
- Jane Iredale eye shadow in Supernova $
- Dr. Hauschka eyeliner in 04 (Espresso Bean) $
- Sukicolor Rich Pigment mascara in Black Velvet $$
- Lumiere Cosmetics blush in Cherry Blossom $
- Sukicolor pure cream stain in Chestnut $$$

NAME: *Konni Corriere*

I love everything about makeup. I love how it changes from year to year. I love the colors and how they change from bright to dark to light to muted to frosted. As the fashions change, so does makeup.

Age: 59

Occupation: Retired psychotherapist

Ethnicity: Caucasian (Norwegian, Scottish, Irish, and English)

Skin Type: Very dry

Relationship status: Divorced

I taught myself how to apply makeup when I was 13. I read through fashion magazines and cut out the looks that I wanted to have, taped them to the mirror, and tried to copy them so that I could look like the pictures.

My skin has certainly changed over the years. Aside from acquiring numerous lines and old-lady wrinkles (as well as some age spots), surprisingly my skin doesn't seem to be as dry as it was when I was younger. However, it's still quite dry.

Being a towhead all my life with pale, shapeless eyebrows and very few lashes, I always went for heavy black eyeliner and thick, gloppy black mascara. It was my hope that the black would contrast with my paleness and bring my face to life. I would like to learn how to apply a makeup look that will bring my eyebrows to life.

How to Apply

When you get older, your skin can lose some of its luster and start to look dull. But using too-heavy makeup will actually make you look older. The ticket to a great makeup look in your fifties is using colors that will brighten your face, rather than create drama. I decided to use brown shades that would complement Konni's blue eyes. Start out by applying a medium brown eye shadow to your eyelids. Blend well up to the crease. Next, wet a thin eyeshadow brush with water and dip it into a dark brown eye shadow. Apply it on your upper and lower lash lines to create definition. Curl your eyelashes and apply several coats of black or brown mascara. Next, define your eyebrows by applying brow mascara to the brows. Add some life to your face by applying a warm, light pink blush to the apples of your cheeks and up and out to your cheekbones. Finish off this look by applying a soft pink lipstick using a lip brush.

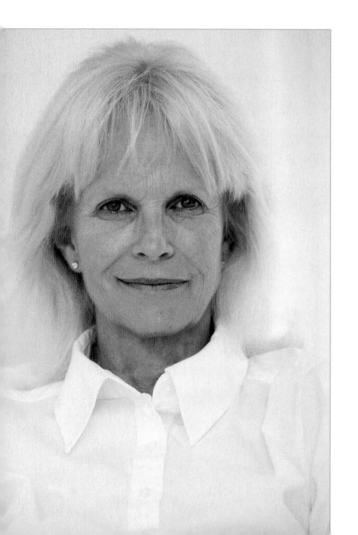

ECO-FRIENDLY PRODUCTS FOR THIS LOOK

- Josie Maran Cosmetics eye shadow in Mist $
- Josie Maran Cosmetics eye shadow in Cappuccino $
- Mineral Fusion Cosmetics lengthening mascara in Rock $
- Jane Iredale PureBrow Gel in Blonde $
- Jane Iredale PurePressed blush in Sheer Honey $$
- Josie Maran Cosmetics lipstick in Flirtatious $

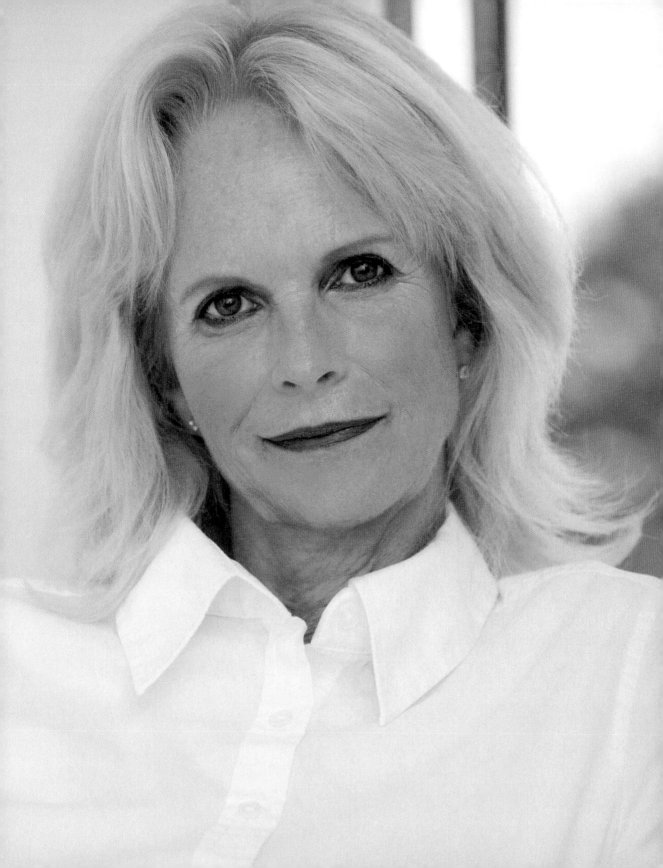

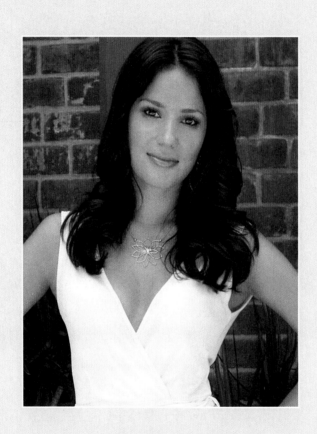

Epilogue

Thank you for joining me on this eco-friendly journey. I hope you enjoyed reading this book as much as I enjoyed writing it. And I hope that you've begun to think more and more about the environment and how you can be eco-beautiful every day.

One thing that's for sure is that we are all creatures of habit. We live busy lives, and time is a precious commodity. When we become accustomed to a product, we tend to stick with it. But it's important to remember that the choices you make on a daily basis don't just affect you, but also the world around you. I'm not asking you to change your entire life tomorrow. But I am suggesting that you make some gradual adjustments as often as you can, and remember to consider the health of our planet when you're about to purchase a product.

The products I've recommended in this book are all widely available. For example, Bare Escentuals and Juice Beauty are sold at Sephora. Mineral Fusion Cosmetics and Dr.Hauschka can be picked up at Whole Foods. Healthier alternatives are out there and at your fingertips. They can be purchased online; you can search the

Internet to find out where they are sold in your area. Once you locate them and incorporate them into your routine, you'll ask yourself why you didn't do it sooner.

There are no shortcuts to becoming healthier, and the only thing stopping you from doing it is . . . you. Take what you have learned in this book, apply your own good judgment, and I promise you'll be on your way and *loving* the results. I certainly did when I made the switch to an eco-beautiful life.

Glossary

Allergen: A substance that can cause a person to have an adverse allergic reaction or hypersensitivity. This substance can be anything from environmental pollution to pet dander to an ingredient in a food or cosmetic product.

Aloe vera: A sticky, gel-like juice extracted from the aloe plant. Applied to the skin, its calming and soothing properties make it extremely helpful for individuals who are suffering from skin irritations and burns.

Alpha lipoic acid: This powerful antioxidant helps prevent cell damage and fights off the aging effects of free-radical damage. It has also been known to reduce the risk of cancer, liver disease, and heart disease. It is popularly taken in pill form, but it can also be found in vegetables like broccoli, spinach, and Brussels sprouts.

Amino acids: These are the "building blocks" of proteins and muscle tissue. Humans have the ability to generate up to 20 amino acids. The others are found in the foods we eat. Since humans can't store amino acids, we also need to get them from our diet. Some examples of amino-rich foods are almonds, soybeans, peanuts, seafood, and tomatoes.

Antioxidant: A substance that protects the cells in the body by neutralizing free radicals, thereby halting the breakdown of collagen and elastin. There are many valuable free-radical-fighting antioxidant substances—such as vitamin A, vitamin B, and beta carotene—that can be found in green tea, pomegranates, blueberries, and other foods.

Blackhead: The small head of a pore clogged by dirt or oil. Blackheads can form when skin hasn't been properly cleaned, thus creating an oil buildup and clogged pores.

Certified organic: A product (usually food- or beauty-related) that is produced using all of the appropriate organic actions and without the use of hormones or pesticides.

The item must meet standard organic requirements to bear the "USDA Certified Organic" logo. Any cosmetic product labeled "Certified Organic" contains 100 percent organic ingredients. Absolutely no synthetic chemicals may be used at any stage of the production chain, including the growing, harvesting, storage, transporting, and processing stages.

Coal tar dye: Dye made from coal tar, which contains harmful toxins and impurities. Coal tar dye can be found in conventional hair dyes and cosmetic products such as lipsticks. It has been shown to produce cancer in laboratory animals.

Collagen: A protein that supports the body's connective tissues. Collagen makes up 75 percent of human skin and is a key component for strength and elasticity. When the skin has sufficient collagen, it appears to be smooth, plump, and youthful.

Detoxification: The process of cleansing the body and its organs by removing unhealthy substances. Many people feel that detoxification promotes feelings of a clearer mind, increases energy, and improves sleep.

DNA (deoxyribonucleic acid): Contains the genetic instructions used in the development and functioning of all living organisms. The sun can adversely affect an individual's skin DNA by altering the enzymes that help repair it.

Elastin: Like collagen, elastin helps support the tissues in the body. This protein surrounds the skin and allows it to stretch, be flexible, and then go back to its normal shape without damage. Without elastin the skin is not nearly as durable.

Enzymes: These are active proteins found in all living things. When it comes to digestion, the human body produces enzymes to break down foods. Healthy enzymes are also found in uncooked raw vegetables and fruits, such as papaya and pineapple.

Epidermis: This is the surface layer of the skin. The epidermis is considered the protective layer of the three layers that make up the skin.

Ester-C: An advanced form of vitamin C, Ester-C is a very powerful antioxidant product that has become quite popular as a means of fighting the appearance of aging skin. This product is often applied to the face in a serum format.

Exfoliation: The process of peeling away and removing dead layers of skin from the face and body. Dead skin cells block the healthy, living skin underneath. Exfoliating can promote vibrant-looking skin.

Flaxseed oil: An important oil for the skin that derives from the ripe seeds of the flax plant. It offers the essential fatty acids omega-3, omega-6, and omega-9. Flaxseed oil also aids the immune, cardiovascular, and reproductive systems, among others. Taking it internally will also help strengthen hair and nails.

Free radicals: Highly reactive and unstable molecules or atoms in the body that cause cellular damage and promote premature aging. Free radicals collide with other molecules in your body to try to steal an electron, and they may damage your DNA and cells in the process. They also can make it hard for the body to fight off infection. Free radicals can be found in processed foods, cigarette smoke, polluted city air, skin that is overexposed to the sun, and elsewhere. Antioxidants are important in helping the body to fight off free radicals.

Gluten: This is a common protein found in many types of bread and cereal products. A person who has an allergy to gluten suffers from what is known as celiac disease. It has been widely reported that a gluten-free diet is helpful for children who suffer from autism.

Grape seed extract: A valuable free-radical fighter, due to its high antioxidant content. Grape seed extract comes from the seeds of red grapes and can be found as an ingredient in various eco-friendly cosmetics products.

Holistic: An approach to health that considers the "whole body" and the "whole person," which includes spiritual and mental needs. Holistic cosmetics and skin-care products are made from all-natural ingredients.

Homeostasis: An internal state of equilibrium in the body. In reference to the skin, homeostasis is when your complexion is completely balanced.

Hormones: Natural chemicals, produced and released within the body, that can affect such processes as metabolism, fertility, growth, immunity, and mood.

Hyaluronic Acid: An acid that occurs naturally in the skin. It absorbs moisture from the air to help lubricate and hydrate the skin. Hyaluronic acid is an important element in the prevention of premature aging.

Hypoallergenic: Products that carry this designation contain ingredients that have little chance of causing an allergic reaction. Hypoallergenic products are manufactured with human allergenic sensitivities in mind and usually are free of perfumes, dyes, and other possible irritants.

Immune system: The body's immune system fights off the viruses, parasites, and bacteria that can make you sick. The defender cells T and B make up the immune system. When it is not running at its optimum level, the skin's complexion can suffer.

Lead: A proven neurotoxin that can cause very serious health problems. Numerous conventional lipsticks contain lead in their formulations.

Meditation: A state of deep and sustained mental relaxation. Meditation frees the mind of distraction and offers the benefits of improved mental clarity and concentration.

Natural products: Products that are developed and made without the addition of synthetic additives like chemical preservatives, colors, or fragrances. The majority of natural cosmetic components are derived from plant extracts and/or natural ingredients.

Nutrition: The process by which living creatures gain energy and vitamins from food and drink for growth, repair, and maintenance. Proper nutrition promotes health and wards off disease.

Olive oil: Derived from pressed tree-ripened olives, olive oil is good for the heart, lowers cholesterol, and helps fight cancer, among other benefits. In addition to its use in cooking, it can also be used externally on the skin.

Omega-3 fatty acids: These are essential fatty acids that are helpful in reducing cholesterol levels and heart disease, as well as in supporting the health of skin, hair, and nails. They also improve the immune system and bone growth. Omega-3 fatty acids can be found in foods such as flaxseeds, salmon, sardines, nuts, and tofu.

Organic products: Products that are made without the use of chemicals, pesticides, hormones, and other harmful ingredients. The materials used in the organic makeup must be from plant material or from substances derived from plant materials, they must be beneficial to the environment, and they must not be genetically modified.

Parabens: Chemicals used as a preservative to prolong the shelf life of conventional moisturizers and makeup products, as well as men's shaving creams and other cosmetics products. Parabens can cause skin irritation, so look for products marked "paraben free."

Petrochemicals: Chemicals that are derived from petroleum, such as ethylene and propylene. They are used in the manufacturing of medicines, plastics, paint, and many other items. They are also found in conventional cosmetic items, including lip gloss and nail polish.

pH balanced: pH is the level of acidity or alkalinity of a solution. If a beauty product is marked "pH balanced" it means the pH levels in the product match the natural pH levels in your body. pH is calculated on a scale of 0 to 14, with 7 being neutral.

Pomegranate: Native to the Middle East, this fruit has extremely high antioxidant properties that are known to help fight aging. This vital fruit is available in juice and pill forms, as well.

Propylene glycol: Used in moisturizers, this substance is derived from petroleum oil and is found in automatic brakes and industrial defrosters. Propylene glycol is toxic and may damage cell membranes, causing redness, rashes, and dry skin. It can also penetrate your skin and enter your bloodstream.

Proteins: These are organic macromolecules that are essential to the body and its ability to grow and repair tissue. Proteins play an important role in building cartilage, as well as in helping to keep the skin firm.

Pycnogenol: A highly powerful antioxidant that is derived from the bark of pine trees. Pycnogenol is a significant ally in the fight against free radicals. It is available in pill form and in various skin-care products.

Recycling: The process by which a product is broken down into its raw materials and readied for reuse.

Rosacea: A skin condition that can cause redness, pimples, and inflammation. It is visible in the form of patches and is usually located on the cheeks, chin, forehead and/or nose.

Sodium lauryl sulphate (SLS): A substance used as a thickener and foaming agent in shampoos, toothpastes, and cleansers, and as a wetting agent in garage floor cleaners, engine and auto degreasers, and auto cleaning products. SLS can dissolve the oils on your skin, which can cause the skin to separate, creating fine lines and wrinkles.

SPF (sun protection factor): The protection number on sunscreens that represents the amount of minutes you can stay in the sun without getting burned. The SPF number on sunscreen products ranges from 2 to 75.

Talc: This soft, mineral, powderlike substance is composed of hydrated magnesium silicate and is used to absorb moisture. Talc is found in cosmetics powders and eye shadows, and long-term use has been reported to cause health problems.

Toxin: A substance that is poisonous and extremely harmful to living organisms.

T-zone: The part of the face consisting of the forehead, nose, and chin. It is often the oiliest part of the face and where many breakouts occur.

Ultraviolet (UV) rays: Electromagnetic light that comes from the sun. Overexposure is a health risk and may lead to skin cancer or sunburn, which can cause redness, itchiness, and inflammation. Skin does absorb the essential vitamin D from ultraviolet exposure, but this vitamin can also be found in some foods, such as oily fish.

Vegan: The practice of a lifestyle that is free of all animal-based products, including milk, meat, cheese, gelatin, eggs, and honey.

Vegetarian: The practice of a meatless and fishless diet. A vegetarian's food intake usually consists of fruits and vegetables, grains, beans, and nuts. Unlike vegans, vegetarians do eat dairy products.

Vitamin A: A vitamin known to improve eyesight and help maintain a healthy heart. Vitamin A comes in the form of retinol and is great for the skin, acting as a powerful wrinkle fighter and helping to fade age spots.

Vitamin B$_5$: This vitamin helps to support your adrenal glands, which regulate your metabolism and help to reduce stress levels. It has been reported that many individuals who suffer from depression have low levels of vitamin B$_5$.

Vitamin C: This is vital for a healthy immune system and it reduces high blood pressure, thus lowering your risk of suffering a stroke. It's also helpful in fighting cancer. Strawberries, oranges, and papaya are great sources of vitamin C.

Vitamin D: A vitamin that is crucial to maintaining healthy bones. Vitamin D wards off osteoporosis, a disease that involves the loss of bone density.

Vitamin E: This is another powerful antioxidant that can help fight premature aging. It also softens and heals the skin from damage. Vitamin E can be taken in pill form, and found in oils such as sunflower oil, soybean oil, and olive oil, as well as in seeds and nuts.

Resources

Eco-Friendly Makeup Companies

Bare Escentuals (bareescentuals.com)

Cargo Cosmetics PlantLove (cargocosmetics.com)

Dr. Hauschka (drhauschka.com)

Ecco Bella (eccobella.com)

Jane Iredale Mineral Cosmetics (janeiredale.com)

Josie Maran Cosmetics (josiemarancosmetics.com)

Lavera Cosmetics (lavera.com)

Lumiere Cosmetics (lumierecosmetics.com)

Miessence (miorganicproducts.com)

Mineral Fusion Cosmetics (mineralfusioncosmetics.com)

Neutrogena Sheer Minerals (neutrogena.com)

Nvey Eco Organics (econveybeauty.com)

Suki (sukipure.com)

Eco-Friendly Skin-Care Companies

Aubrey Organics (aubrey-organics.com)

Aveda (aveda.com)

Burt's Bees (burtsbees.com)

Desert Essence (desertessence.com)

Dr.Hauschka (drhauschka.com)

Éminence Organics (eminenceorganics.com)

Jason Natural (jason-natural.com)

Juice Beauty (juicebeauty.com)

Jurlique Skin Care (jurlique.com)

Lavera (lavera.com)

Miessence (miorganicproducts.com)

mod.skin labs (modskinlabs.com)

MyChelle Dermaceuticals (mychelleusa.com)

Stella McCartney (stellamccartneycare.com)

Suki (sukipure.com)

Weleda (usa.weleda.com)

Eco-Friendly Makeup Tool Companies

EcoTools (parispresents.com)

Lumiere Cosmetics (lumierecosmetics.com)

Mineral Fusion Cosmetics (mineralfusioncosmetics.com)

Suki (sukipure.com)

Tweezerman (tweezerman.com)

Green Web Sites

Be Green (begreennow.com)

Earth 911 (earth911.com)

EcoStiletto (ecostiletto.com)

Green Guide (thegreenguide.com)

Green Living (greenlivingonline.com)

Green Your (greenyour.com)

Grist (grist.org)

Green Shopping Web Sites

Ecomall (ecomall.com)

Gaiam (gaiam.com)

GreenDeals Daily (greendealsdaily.com)

Greenfeet (greenfeet.com)

Green Home (greenhome.com)

GreenShopper (greenshopper.com)

Greenzer (greenzer.com)

So Organic (soorganic.com)

Green Blogs

EarthFirst (earthfirst.com)

Eco Chick (eco-chick.com)

EcoGeek (ecogeek.org)

Greenthinkers (greenthinkers.org)

Groovy Green (groovygreen.com)

Ideal Bite (idealbite.com)

Lighter Footstep (lighterfootstep.com)

TreeHugger (treehugger.com)

True Green Confessions (truegreenconfessions.com)

Books for an Eco-Friendly Lifestyle, Beauty, and Wellness

MacEachern, Diane. *Big Green Purse: Use Your Spending Power to Create a Cleaner, Greener World.* New York, NY: Avery, 2008.

Loux, Renee. *Easy Green Living: The Ultimate Guide to Simple, Eco-Friendly Choices for You and Your Home.* Emmaus, PA: Rodale, 2008.

Taylor, Nancy H. and Gibbs Smith. *Go Green: How to Build an Earth-Friendly Community.* Layton, UT: 2008.

Uliano, Sophie. *Gorgeously Green: 8 Simple Steps to an Earth-Friendly Life.* New York, NY: Collins Living, 2008.

Rogers, Elizabeth and Thomas M. Kostigen. *The Green Book: The Everyday Guide to Saving the Planet One Simple Step at a Time.* New York, NY: Three Rivers Press, 2007.

Matheson, Christie. *Green Chic: Saving the Earth in Style.* Naperville, IL: Sourcebooks, 2008.

Trask, Crissy and Gibbs Smith. *It's Easy Being Green: A Handbook for Earth-Friendly Living.* Layton, UT: Gibbs Smith. 2006.

Dorfman, Josh. *The Lazy Environmentalist: Your Guide to Easy, Stylish, Green Living.* New York, NY: Stewart, Tabori & Chang, 2007.

Begley, Ed Jr. *Living Like Ed: A Guide to the Eco-Friendly Life.* New York, NY: Clarkson Potter, 2008.

Tourles, Stephanie. *Organic Body Care Recipes: 175 Homemade Herbal Formulas for Glowing Skin and a Vibrant Self.* North Adams, MA: Storey, 2007.

Freston, Kathy. *Quantum Wellness: A Practical and Spiritual Guide to Health and Happiness.* New York, NY: Weinstein Books, 2008.

Eby, Myra Michelle with Karolyn A. Gazella. *Return to Beautiful Skin: Your Guide to Truly Effective, Nontoxic Skin Care.* Laguna Beach, CA: Basic Health, 2008.

Hagen, Annelise. *The Yoga Face: Eliminate Wrinkles with the Ultimate Natural Facelift.* New York, NY: Avery, 2007.

Books For Healthy Eating, Drinking, and Living

Wolfe, David. *Eating for Beauty.* San Diego, CA: North Atlantic Books, 2003.

O'Brien, Susan. *Gluten-free, Sugar-free Cooking: Over 200 Delicious Recipes to Help You Live a Healthier, Allergy-Free Life.* New York, NY: Da Capo, 2006.

Boutenko, Victoria. *Green for Life.* Ashland, OR: Raw Family Publishing, 2005.

Orey, Cal. *The Healing Powers of Olive Oil: A Complete Guide to Nature's Liquid Gold.* New York, NY: Kensington, 2009.

Bailey, Steven ND, and Larry Trivieri, Jr. *Juice Alive: The Ultimate Guide to Juicing Remedies.* Garden City Park, NY: Square, 2006.

Blauer, Stephen. *The Juicing Book: A Complete Guide to the Juicing of Fruits and Vegetables for Maximum Health and Vitality.* New York, NY: Avery, 1989.

Underkoffler, Renee Loux. *Living Cuisine: The Art and Spirit of Raw Foods.* New York, NY: Avery, 2004.

Kenney, Matthew and Sarma Melngailis. *Raw Food/Real World: 100 Recipes to Get the Glow.* New York, NY: William Morrow Cookbooks, 2005.

Barkie, Karen E. *Sweet and Sugar Free: An All-Natural Fruit-Sweetened Dessert Cookbook.* New York, NY: St. Martin's Griffin, 1982.

Blereau, Jude. *Wholefood: 300 Recipes to Restore, Nourish, and Delight.* Philadelphia, PA: Running Press, 2007.

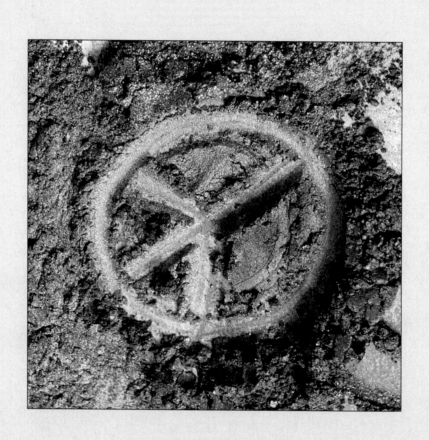

About the Author

Makeup artist **Lina Hanson** was born in Stockholm, Sweden. Lina later moved to London, England, where she began working in the fashion industry. She then relocated to New York City to pursue her true passion— a career as a makeup artist.

Lina has since established a distinct image for herself in the makeup industry. She has created red-carpet looks for events such as the Academy Awards, Golden Globes, Grammys, and Emmys. Her skilled artistry has appeared in *Vogue, W, Harper's Bazaar, InStyle, Interview,* and *Elle.* She is represented by the Magnet Agency and lives in Los Angeles.

For more information about Lina, visit her Web site at linahanson.com.

Dove Shore is a photographer whose images express a wide range of interests. From the runways of the fashion world, to the urban streets of Los Angeles, to the banks of the Ganges in India, his work reflects a true engagement from one side of the lens to the other. His photography has appeared in *Elle, Rolling Stone, InStyle, Entertainment Weekly* and *The New York Times*.

Dove lives in Los Angeles. For more information visit his Web site doveshore.com

---

Mara Roszak grew up in the Laurel Canyon area of Los Angeles. At 17, Mara graduated from beauty school and was hired to work at the prestigious Chris McMillan Salon. Mara's client list is extensive, having worked with Halle Berry, Elisha Cuthbert, Sarah Michelle Gellar, and Amanda Bynes, among others. She has also worked with many publications, most notably *Flaunt, Esquire, British Esquire, Hollywood Life,* and *Cosmo Girl*. Mara currently works at the Byron Salon in Beverly Hills.

Index

Boldface page references indicate photographs. Underscored references indicate boxed text.

A

Acne
- coconut water for, 31
- conventional shaving products and, 99
- dehydration and, 29
- dirty makeup brushes and, 13
- expired makeup and, 70
- oily skin and, 43
- shaving cream and, 99

Adrenal glands, 26

Aftershave, 102, 104

Agave nectar, 32

Agency for Toxic Substances and Disease Registry (ATSDR), 10

Aging. *See also* Wrinkles
- eco-friendly cosmetic products in fighting, 16
- free radicals and, 16, 20
- makeup and
  - changes in, 146
  - fifties, 159–60, **160**, 160, **161**
  - forties, 156, **156**, **157**, 158, 158
  - teens, 147–48, **148**, 148, **149**
  - thirties, 153–54, **154**, 154, **155**
  - twenties, 150, **150**, **151**, 152, 152
- minimizing
  - cinnamon, 33
  - diet, 20–21
  - herbs, 33
  - spices, 33
- sun exposure and, 56

Aguacate & Co. Facial Exfoliating Crème, 102

Airplane travel, 27

Air pollution, indoor, 35

Alba Botanica Organic Lavender, 110

Allergies, skin, 57, 108

Almond milk
- Berry Blast juice, 37

Almond oil for body lotion, 93

Almonds for exfoliation, 50

Almond-shaped eyes, 79

Aloe for sunburn, 59

American Botanical Council study, 20

Animal-friendly products. *See also* Eco-friendly cosmetic products
- makeup brushes, 13
- shaving, 100

Anthocyanins, 21

Antioxidants, 2, 20

Apple cider vinegar for toning skin, 53

Applying makeup. *See also* Aging, makeup and; Daytime makeup; Eye shadow; Lipstick; Nighttime makeup; Seasonal makeup
- blush, 73–74, 74
- bronzer, 75–76, 75
- clean, healthy skin before starting, 66–67
- eye shadow, 76–80, 77, 78, 79
- foundation
  - concealer, 70–71, 71
  - cream, 68, 68
  - liquid, 67–68, 67
  - mineral, 69, 69
  - setting powder, 72, 72
  - switching out, 70
  - tinted moisturizer, 67–68, 67, 85

Applying makeup *(cont.)*
 lighting for, <u>83</u>
 lipstick, 86–88, **87**, <u>88</u>
 mascara, 80–81, **80**, <u>80</u>
 at office, <u>115</u>
 self-knowledge and, 65–66
Arcona
 Cool Zone facial hydrator, 106
 Cranberry Gommage, 46
 Golden Grain Gommage, 52
 Kiwi Cream, 107
 Magic White Ice hydrating gel, 49
 Reozone full-spectrum sunscreen, <u>58</u>
 Triad Pads for Men, <u>107</u>
Arcona Studio, <u>60</u>
Artichokes for healthy skin, 21
Artificial sweeteners, 32
ATSDR, 10
Aubrey Organics
 Blue Green Algae facial toner, 49, 53
 facial cleansing lotion, 47
 Jojoba Meal & Oatmeal mask and scrub, 50
 Men's Stock cleansing bar, 106
 Men's Stock moisturizer, 106
 Natural Sun Green Tea sunscreen, <u>58</u>
 Rosa Mosqueta rose hip moisturizing cream, 51
Aveda Men After-Shave Balm, <u>102</u>
Awww-tumn fall look, 138, <u>138</u>, **139**

B

Baking soda
 for callus removal, <u>89</u>
 for exfoliation, <u>52</u>
Bare Escentuals bareMinerals
 All-Over face color, <u>74</u>
 blush, <u>148</u>
 cheek color, <u>141</u>
 eye shadow, <u>78</u>, <u>79</u>, <u>118</u>

liner shadow, <u>123</u>
 100% Natural lip color, <u>88</u>
 SPF 15 foundation, <u>69</u>
Bath for relaxation, 54
Beans for healthy skin, 21
Beetroot for healthy skin, 21
Beta-carotene, 21, 32
Blackberries
 Berry Blast juice, 37
Blackheads, 43. *See also* Acne
Black skin tone, 74
Blemishes. *See* Acne
Bliss Mix by Transition Nutrition, <u>22</u>
Blood-sugar levels, <u>22</u>, 32
Blueberries
 Berry Blast juice, 37
 for healthy skin, 21–22
Blue eyes, 78
Blush, 73–74, <u>74</u>, 84. *See also specific product*
Body lotion, homemade, 93
Body type and diet, 20
Bronze/dark skin tone, 73
Bronzed Babe look, 122, **123**, <u>123</u>
Bronzer, 75–76, <u>75</u>
Brown eyes, 76
Brown rice for healthy skin, 22
Burt's Bees
 Natural Skin Care for Men, 106
 Res-Q Ointment, <u>55</u>
Business Chic look, **118**, <u>118</u>, 119
B vitamins, 22, 33

C

Caffeine
 in coffee, 26
 side effects of, 26
 skin and, 26–28
Calcium, 21, 23, 32

Callus remover remedy, <u>89</u>

Cancer, skin, 42, 56, 108

Carbohydrates, 22

Cargo PlantLove lipstick, 12, <u>12</u>, <u>88</u>

Castor oil for eye makeup remover, 91

Cayenne, 34

Celery

    All Green juice, 36

Certified organic cosmetic products, 5–7

CFCs, 99–100

CFLs, <u>83</u>

Chamomile

    for cleansing skin, <u>50</u>

    for toning skin, <u>53</u>

Changes to personal appearance,
    need for, 15

Chapped skin, 43

Chemical Safe Skincare Campaign, 10

Chlorofluorocarbons (CFCs), 99–100

Cinnamon, 33–34

Cleansing. *See also specific product*

    chamomile for, <u>50</u>

    combination skin, 52, <u>52</u>

    cucumbers for, <u>48</u>

    dry skin, 50, <u>50</u>

    lemons for, <u>48</u>

    for men, 105–7, <u>107</u>

    normal skin, 46, <u>46</u>

    oily skin, 48, <u>48</u>

    organic cream for, <u>50</u>

    organic milk for, <u>46</u>, <u>50</u>

    yogurt for, <u>52</u>

Coal tar dyes, avoiding, 11

Coconut oil, 25–26

Coconuts, 31

Coconut water, 30–31

Coffee

    caffeine in, 26

    decaffeinated, 27

    dehydration and, 26

    skin and, 26–28

    substitute for, <u>27</u>, 28

Collagen

    beetroot in promoting, 21

    gender differences, 97

    sugar and, 31

Color

    of eyes, 76–79

    seasonal, 137, <u>137</u>

Combination skin

    cleansing, 52, <u>52</u>

    defining, 43

    exfoliating, 52, <u>52</u>

    moisturizing, 53

    toning, 53, <u>53</u>

Compact fluorescent lightbulbs (CFLs), <u>83</u>

Concealer, 70–71, <u>71</u>. *See also specific product*

Conservation movement, 1

Conventional cosmetic products, 5, 10

Cool Chick winter look, **140**, 141, <u>141</u>

Corriere, Konni, 159, <u>159</u>, **160**, **161**

Cortese, Genevieve, <u>150</u>, <u>150</u>, **151**

Cracked skin, 43

Cranberries for healthy skin, 22

Cream blush, 74, <u>74</u>, 84

Cream eye shadow, 84–85

Cream foundation, 68, <u>68</u>

Cucumbers

    All Green juice, 36

    for cleansing skin, <u>48</u>

    for sunburn, 59

Cuts on skin, <u>55</u>

D

D'Amato, Kim, 89

Dandy Blend, <u>27</u>, 28

Dark circles under eyes, <u>59</u>

Dark spots on skin, 56

Daytime makeup
    appropriate, 114
    Bronzed Babe look, 122, **123**, <u>123</u>
    Business Chic look, **118**, <u>118</u>, 119
    eye shadow, 76–79
    Fun and Flirty look, 120, **121**, <u>121</u>
    No-Makeup Makeup Look, 116, **117**, <u>117</u>
    types of looks, 115
DBP, avoiding, 89
Decaffeinated coffee, 27
Dehydration
    acne and, 29
    coffee and, 26
    hot water and, <u>44</u>
Desert Essence Organics, 55
Detoxification, 23, 30
Dibutyl phthalate (DBP), avoiding, 89
Diet. *See also specific food*
    anti-aging, 20–21
    antioxidant-rich, 20
    body type and, 20
    carbohydrates in, 22
    coconut water and, 30–31
    coffee, 26–28
    fiber in, <u>22</u>, 23, 32, 35
    fruits, 35
    hair health and, 21
    herbs, 33–34
    juices, 34–35
    oils, 24–26
    protein in, 21, 31
    skin and, 20–23
    spices, 33–34
    sugar, 31–33
    vegetables, <u>20</u>, 35
    water intake and, 29–30
Digestion, 30
Diuretic, 26

Dr. Hauschka
    bronzing powder, <u>75</u>
    eyeliner, <u>127</u>, <u>131</u>, <u>158</u>
    eye shadow, <u>77</u>, <u>78</u>
    facial toner, 47
    Kajal eyeliner, <u>121</u>
    lipstick, <u>132</u>
    liquid concealer, <u>71</u>
    liquid eyeliner, <u>132</u>
    Novum lip gloss, <u>88</u>, <u>148</u>
    rouge powder, <u>74</u>, <u>145</u>
    translucent makeup, <u>67</u>
    Volume mascara, <u>81</u>, <u>117</u>, <u>121</u>, <u>142</u>, <u>145</u>
Dry skin
    cleansing, 50, <u>50</u>
    defining, 43
    effects of, 96–97
    exfoliating, 50, <u>50</u>
    in men, 96–97, 107
    moisturizing, 51
    olive oil for, 24–25
    toning, 51, <u>51</u>

E

Ecco Bella
    FlowerColor, face powder, <u>72</u>
    FlowerColor bronzing powder, <u>75</u>
    FlowerColor lipstick, <u>88</u>
    FlowerColor natural liquid foundation, <u>67</u>
    FlowerColor natural mascara, <u>128</u>, <u>132</u>, <u>148</u>, <u>154</u>
    Mist-On Toner, 51
    soft eyeliner pencil, <u>128</u>
"Eco-application", 66. *See also* Applying makeup
Eco-friendly cosmetic products. *See also* Applying makeup; *specific product*

for animal lovers, 13, 17

anti-aging effects of, 16

antioxidants in, 2

availability of, 163–64

benefits of using, 2, 4, 16–17

cost of, 16, _66_

doing good and, 16

expired, avoiding, _70_

health and, commitment to, 17

homemade

    body lotion, 93

    eye makeup remover, 91

    fun of, 91

    lip balm, 92

Maran's views on, 8–9

new look and, 15

at office, _115_

pregnant women and, 10–11, 17

transitioning to, 15–16

types of, 4–7

varieties of, 4

vitamins in, 2, 17

Eco-friendly hair products, _104_

Eco-friendly skin products, 42, 44, 57

Eco-friendly sunscreen products,
    110–11

Eco Lips Organic Sport lip balm, 110

EcoTools, 13, 75, _82_

Eczema, 41

EGF, 106

Eggs, healthy hair and raw, _32_

Egg yolk for body lotion, 93

Electrolytes, 31

Energy and water intake, 29–30

Environmental Protection Agency (EPA),
    98–99

Envirosax, _21_

EPA, 98–99

Epidermal growth factor (EGF), 106

Essential oils

    for body lotion, 93

    for lip balm, 92

Exfoliation. _See also specific product_

    almonds for, _50_

    baking soda for, _52_

    combination skin, 52, _52_

    dry skin, 50, _50_

    lemon juice for, _48_

    mayonnaise for, _50_

    normal skin, 46, _46_

    oatmeal for, _46_, _52_

    oily skin, 48, _48_

    sea salt for, _48_

    yogurt for, _46_

Expired makeup, avoiding, _70_

Eyebrows

    importance of, 81

    maintaining, 81–83

    shaping

        tips for, _82_, _83_

        tools for, _82_

Eyebrow tools, _82_

Eye makeup remover, homemade, 91

Eyes

    almond-shaped, 79

    blue, 78

    brown, 76

    color of, 76–79

    dark circles under, _59_

    eyebrows

        importance of, 81

        maintaining, 81–83

        tips for shaping, _82_, _83_

        tools for shaping, _82_

    eye shadow

        almond-shaped eyes, 79

        applying, 76–80, _77_, _78_, _79_

        blue eyes, 78, _78_

Eyes
    eye shadow *(cont.)*
        brown eyes, 77, _77_
        color of eyes and, 76–77
        daytime makeup, 76–79
        green eyes, 78, _78_
        hazel eyes, 79, _79_
        importance of, 76
        recycling cream, 84–85
        small eyes, 80
        wide-set eyes, 79
    hazel, 79
    heavy makeup tips, _137_
    small, 80
    wide-set, 79
Eye shadow
    almond-shaped eyes, 79
    applying, 76–80, _77_, _78_, _79_
    blue eyes, 78, _78_
    brown eyes, 77, _77_
    color of eyes and, 76–77
    cream, 84–85
    daytime makeup, 76–79
    green eyes, 78, _78_
    hazel eyes, 79, _79_
    importance of, 76
    recycling cream, 84–85
    small eyes, 80
    wide-set eyes, 79

F

Facial features, 76
Facial mist, _43_
Facials, 60–63
Fall makeup look, 138, _138_, **139**
Fiber, _22_, 23, 32, 35
Fifties makeup look, 159–60, **160**, _160_, **161**
Fish, _57_

Fish oil, 25
Flaxseed oil, 25
Foot care, 89, _89_, _111_
Formaldehyde, avoiding, 89
Forties makeup look, 156, **156**, **157**, 158, _158_
Foundation. *See also specific product*
    concealer, 70–71, _71_
    cream, 68, _68_
    liquid, 67–68, _67_
    mineral, 69, _69_
    setting powder, 72, _72_
    switching out, _70_
    tinted moisturizer, 67–68, _67_, 85
Fragrances, avoiding synthetic, _17_
Free radicals
    aging and, 16, 20
    papaya in preventing damage from, _107_
    prevalence of, 2
Freshening makeup, _115_, _125_
Fruits, 35. *See also specific type*
Fun and Flirty look, 120, **121**, _121_

G

Garlic, 34
Gillette, _100_
Ginger, 34
Gingerroot
    Immune Zoom juice, 38
Glamour Girl look, **132**, _132_, 133
"Go Green" Mini Slant tweezer, _82_
Goji berries
    Berry Blast juice, 37
    for healthy skin, 22–23
Grapeseed oil for eye makeup remover, 91
"Greek glow," 24
Green-Carpet Ready look, **128**, _128_, 129
Green eyes, 78, _78_
"Green" movement, 1

H

Habit, humans as creatures of, 15
Hair care and health
    coconut water and, 31
    diet and, 21
    eco-friendly products, <u>104</u>
    eggs, raw, <u>32</u>
    for men, <u>104</u>
    olive oil and, <u>32</u>
Hanson, Lina, 19–20, 113–14, 135–36,
    162, 163–64
Harrelson, Woody, <u>100</u>
Hazel eyes, 79
Herbs, 33–34. *See also specific type*
High blood pressure, <u>28</u>
Hollywood celebrities, 1
Honey, 32–33
Hot Stuff summer look, **144**, 145,
    <u>145</u>
Hot water and dehydration, <u>44</u>
Hourglass Cosmetics, 13
Houseplants, <u>35</u>
Hyaluronic acid, 21
Hypertension, <u>28</u>

I

Insulin levels, 31
Iron, 21, <u>22</u>
Ivory/light beige skin tone, 73

J

Jane Iredale
    Active Light under-eye concealer, <u>71</u>
    Amazing Base loose mineral foundation,
    <u>69</u>
    blush, <u>121</u>
    Circle/Delete under-eye concealer,
    <u>71</u>
    eye highlighter pencil, <u>141</u>, <u>145</u>
    eye shadow, <u>138</u>, <u>158</u>
    In Touch cream blush stick,
    <u>74</u>
    lip pencil, <u>132</u>
    matte powder, <u>72</u>
    PureBrow gel, <u>132</u>, <u>160</u>
    PureGloss, <u>145</u>
    PurePressed blush, <u>74</u>, <u>138</u>, <u>160</u>
    PurePressed triple eye shadow,
    <u>77</u>, <u>78</u>, <u>79</u>, <u>123</u>, <u>142</u>, <u>152</u>
Jason 6-in-1 Beard and Skin Therapy
    shaving lotion, 100
Jason Natural Cosmetics Chemical Free
    sunblock, <u>58</u>
Jenae, Chanel, 60–63, **61**
Josie Maran Cosmetics
    Argan Oil, <u>9</u>
    bronzing powder, <u>75</u>
    concealer, <u>71</u>
    cream blush, <u>74</u>
    eye liner, <u>117</u>, <u>138</u>
    eye shadow, <u>78</u>, <u>127</u>, <u>131</u>, <u>145</u>,
    <u>154</u>, <u>160</u>
    lip gloss, <u>88</u>, <u>117</u>, <u>141</u>
    lipstick, <u>118</u>, <u>128</u>, <u>138</u>, <u>160</u>
    Maran and, 8–9
    mascara, <u>81</u>, <u>131</u>, <u>141</u>, <u>152</u>
    pressed powder, <u>72</u>
    tinted moisturizer, <u>67</u>
Juice Beauty Mineral Sheer moisturizer,
    <u>58</u>
Juices
    All Green, 36
    Berry Blast, 37
    Immune Zoom, 38
    skin and, 34–35

K

Kale
    All Green juice, 36
    for healthy skin, 23
Kiss My Face
    Cell Mate 15 facial cream and sunscreen, 58
    Fragrance Free Moisture Shave, 100
Knudson, Coco, 147, 147, **148**, **149**
Korres
    Magnolia cleansing and moisturizing
        emulsion, 46
    Orange Blossom cleansing and moisturizing
        emulsion, 52

L

Labels
    cosmetic product, 6, 10–11
    food, 6, 10
    shaving cream, 101
Lavera
    lipstick, 88
    Men Care moisturizer, 107
Lemon juice
    for body lotion, 93
    for exfoliation, 48
Lemons
    for cleansing skin, 48
    Immune Zoom juice, 38
Lettuce wraps for sunburn, 59
Lifestyle, healthy, 19–20
Lighting for applying makeup, 83
Lip balm, 92, 110. *See also specific product*
Lip gloss, 84, 88, 88. *See also specific product*
Lipstick. *See also specific product*
    applying, 86–88, **87**, 88
    color, choosing, 86–87
    conventional, 10

    drinking from straw to avoid messing, 124
    lead content in, 10
    matte, 87–88, 88
    recycled, 84
    sheer, 88, 88
    skin and, 86–87
Liquid foundation, 67–68, 67
Litt, Anne, 156, **156**, 156, **157**
Loose minerals blush, 74, 74
L'Oréal, 15
Lowest Flow Showerhead by Real Goods, 30
Lumiere Cosmetics
    blush, 152, 158
    Ditto eye color, 141
    eye pigment, 127, 128, 138, 158
    eye shadow, 77, 78
    face and body enhancer, 123, 128
    lip gloss, 127
    loose mineral foundation, 69
    mineral blush, 74

M

Magnesium, 21
Makeup. *See also* Applying makeup
    aging and
        changes in, 146
        fifties, 159–60, **160**, 160, **161**
        forties, 156, **156**, **157**, 158, 158
        teens, 147–48, **148**, 148, **149**
        thirties, 153–54, **154**, 154, **155**
        twenties, 150, **150**, 151, 152, 152
    expired, avoiding, 70
    freshening, 115, 125
    new look and, 15
Makeup brushes
    cleaning, 13, 14
    dirty, 13–14
    eco-friendly, 13–14, 74

Manicure, 89, <u>111</u>

Maple syrup, organic, 33

Maran, Josie, 8–9

Mascara, 80–81, **80**, <u>80</u>

Mascara wand, <u>85</u>

Matte lipstick, 87–88, <u>88</u>

Maybelline, 8

Mayonnaise for exfoliation, <u>50</u>

Medium/light olive skin tone, 73

Melanoma, 56

Men's grooming issues

    appeal to women and, 95, <u>111</u>

    hair care, <u>104</u>

    for outdoorsman, 108, <u>108</u>

    shaving

        aftershave, <u>102</u>, 104

        frequency of, 98

        olive oil for, <u>103</u>

        post-shave, <u>102</u>, 103–4

        pre-shave, 101–3

        products, 99–103, <u>101</u>

        razors, 98–99

        shaving cream, 99–100, <u>101</u>

        technique, 103

    skin

        cleansing, 105–7, <u>107</u>

        dry, 96–97, 107

        gender differences, 97–98

        normal, 106

        oily, 106

        problems, 96–97

    sun protection, 108, <u>108</u>, 110–11

    trends in, 95–96

Metallic Maven look, 125–26, **127**, <u>127</u>

Miessence

    Balancing moisturiser, 53

    Certified Organic purifying skin cleanser, 48

Milk

    almond, 37

    for cleansing skin, organic, <u>46</u>, <u>50</u>

Mineral cosmetic products, 4–5

Mineral foundation, 69, <u>69</u>

Mineral Fusion Cosmetics

    blush, <u>118</u>, <u>123</u>, <u>131</u>, <u>142</u>, <u>154</u>

    bronzer, <u>75</u>

    concealer, <u>71</u>

    eye pencil, <u>142</u>, <u>148</u>, <u>152</u>

    eye shadow, <u>117</u>, <u>118</u>, <u>154</u>

    lengthening mascara, <u>81</u>, <u>160</u>

    lip gloss, <u>123</u>, <u>152</u>, <u>154</u>

    lip sheer, <u>88</u>

    lipstick, <u>88</u>, <u>142</u>

    setting powder, <u>72</u>

    sheer tint base, <u>67</u>

Minerals, 31. *See also specific type*

Mint leaves for toning skin, <u>51</u>

Mod.Skin Lab

    I.D. Zyne DMAE & Blue Green

        Algae, <u>59</u>

    Samurai Scrub Rice & Enzyme face

        polish, 48

Moisturizer. *See also specific product*

    for combination skin, 53

    for dry skin, 51

    in fall, <u>138</u>

    for men, 106–7

    for normal skin, 47

    for oily skin, 49

    skin changes and, <u>43</u>

    sunburn and, avoiding, 58

    with sunscreen, 57

    tinted, 67–68, <u>67</u>, 85

Moles, 56

Monavé

    blush, <u>74</u>

    loose mineral foundation, <u>69</u>

    mineral cream foundation, <u>68</u>

MyChelle

    cream foundation, <u>68</u>

    Fruit Enzyme Mist, <u>43</u>

N

Nail health and care
    for men, 111
    for women, 31, 89–90
Nail polish, 89–90, 145
Natural cosmetic products, 2, 6–7, 17
Natura Organic Sleep Mask, 84
Neutrogena eye shadow, 78
Nighttime makeup
    appropriate, 114, 124
    eye shadow, 76–79
    freshening makeup and, 125
    Glamour Girl look, **132**, 132, 133
    Green-Carpet Ready look, **128**,
        128, 129
    Metallic Maven look, 125–26, **127**,
        127
    Sexy Vixen look, 130, **131**, 131
No-Makeup Makeup Look, 116, **117**,
    117
Nordic Naturals Ultimate Omega fish
    oil, 25
Normal skin
    cleansing, 46, 46
    defining, 42
    exfoliating, 46, 46
    men's, 106
    moisturizing, 47
    toning, 47, 47
Nvey Eco
    organic compact powder, 72
    organic crème deluxe foundation, 68
    organic eye shadow, 77, 148
    organic lip lustre, 88
    organic liquid foundation, 67
    organic moisturizing mascara,
        118
    organic powder blush, 74

O

Oatmeal
    for breakfast, 22
    for exfoliation, 46, 52
    for sunburn, 59
Office, freshening makeup at, 115
Oils and skin, 24–26
Oily skin
    acne and, 43
    cleansing, 48, 48
    defining, 43
    exfoliating, 48, 48
    men's, 106
    moisturizing, 49
    pregnant women and, 43
    toning, 49, 49
Olive oil
    for body lotion, 93
    for dry skin, 24–25
    for hair care, 32
    for lip balm, 92
    for shaving, 103
Omega-3 fatty acids, 24–25
O.N.E. drink, 31
Oranges
    Immune Zoom juice, 38
Oregano, 34
Organic cosmetic products, 5–6, 50
Organic cream for cleansing skin, 50
Organic extra-virgin olive oil, 24–25
Organic maple syrup, 33
Organic milk for cleansing skin, 46, 50

P

Packaging for cosmetic products, 12
Papaya for cleansing skin, 107

Parabens, avoiding, 11, <u>17</u>, <u>43</u>
Parsley
    All Green juice, 36
Peacekeeper Nail Paint, 90
Pedicure, 89, <u>89</u>, <u>111</u>
PETA-friendly products
    makeup brushes, 13
    shaving, <u>100</u>
Phthalates, avoiding, <u>17</u>
Physicians Formula Organic Wear 100% Natural
    Origin bronzer, <u>75</u>
Pimples. *See* Acne
Pistachio Foot Repair Cream, 55
PlantLove lipstick, 12, <u>12</u>
Plastic shopping bags, avoiding, <u>21</u>
Plastic water bottles, 20
Polished Mama Nail Polish, 90
Pollutants, indoor, <u>35</u>
Post-shave, <u>102</u>, 103–4
Potassium, 23, 32
Pregnant women, 10–11, 17, 43
Preservatives, avoiding, <u>17</u>
Preserve Triple Razor, 99
Pre-shave, 101–3
Priti
    Nail Polish, 90
    Organic Spa, 89
Propylene glycol, avoiding, 11
Protein, 21, 31
Prunes for healthy skin, 23

R

Raspberries
    Berry Blast juice, 37
Razors, 98–99
Recyclable paper and packaging, 12
Recycled air on airplanes, <u>27</u>

Recycling makeup, 84–85
Rosacea, 4
Rosemary, 34
Rose oil for toning, <u>53</u>
Rose water for toning skin, <u>47</u>
Ruberto, Raffaele, <u>17</u>

S

Salt, <u>28</u>, <u>89</u>
Santa Verde Aloe Vera Sunscreen, <u>58</u>
Sea salt for exfoliation, <u>48</u>
Seasonal makeup
    Awww-tumn fall look, 138, <u>138</u>, **139**
    colors for, 137, <u>137</u>
    Cool Chick winter look, **140**, 141, <u>141</u>
    heavy eye makeup tips and, <u>137</u>
    Hot Stuff summer look, **144**, 145, <u>145</u>
    importance of, 136–37
    Spring Fling spring look, 142, <u>142</u>, **143**
Sensatia Botanicals, 54
Setting powder, 72, <u>72</u>
Sexy Vixen look, 130, **131**, <u>131</u>
Shaving
    aftershave, <u>102</u>, 104
    frequency of, 98
    olive oil for, <u>103</u>
    post-shave, <u>102</u>, 103–4
    pre-shave, 101–3
    products, 99–103, <u>101</u>
    razors, 98–99
    shaving cream, 99–101, <u>101</u>
    technique, 103
Shaving cream, 99–101, <u>101</u>
Shea butter for lip balm, 92
Sheer lipstick, 88, <u>88</u>
Showers, taking shorter, 2, <u>30</u>
SIGG reusable water bottle, 30

Singh, Ansu, 153, <u>153</u>, **154**, **155**

Skin. *See also* Acne; *specific type*; Wrinkles

  aging and, 56

  allergies, 57, 108

  bath for relaxation and, 54

  caffeine and, 26–28

  cancer, 42, 56, 108

  challenges of maintaining healthy, 41

  changes to, <u>43</u>

  chapped, 43

  coconut water and, 30–31

  coffee and, 26–28

  cracked, 43

  cuts on, <u>55</u>

  diet and, 20–23

  eco-friendly products, 42, 44, 57

  facials and, 60–63

  foods for healthy

    artichokes, 21

    beans, 21

    beetroot, 21

    blueberries, 21–22

    brown rice, 22

    cranberries, 22

    goji berries, 22–23

    kale, 23

    prunes, 23

    sweet potatoes, 23

  gender differences in, 97–98

  herbs and, 33–34

  hot water and, avoiding, <u>44</u>

  juices and, 34–35

  lipstick and, 86–87

  men's

    cleansing, 105–7, <u>107</u>

    dry, 96–97, 107

    gender differences, 97–98

    normal, 106

    oily, 106

    problems, 96–97

  moles on, 56

  oils and, 24–26

  problems

    conventional cosmetics and, 10

    cuts, <u>55</u>

    dark spots, 56

    eczema, 41

    for men, 96–97

    rosacea, 4

    sunburn, 58–59

  spices and, 33–34

  stress and, 22

  sugar and, 31–33

  sun protection and, 56–57, <u>57</u>

  tips for beautiful, <u>63</u>

  tone

    black, 74

    bronze/dark, 73

    ivory/light beige, 73

    medium/light olive, 73

  types

    combination, 43

    dry, 43

    normal, 42

    oil, 43

  vitamin E and, <u>24</u>

  water intake and, 29–30

Skin Cancer Foundation, 56

Skin products, 42, 44

Sleep tips, <u>84</u>

SLS, avoiding, 11

Small eyes, 80

Snacks, healthy, <u>22</u>

Sodium, <u>28</u>, <u>89</u>

Sodium lauryl sulphate (SLS), avoiding, 11

Soléo Organics sunscreen, 111

Sol Shaver Solar Razor, 99

Spices, 33–34. *See also specific type*

Spinach

  All Green juice, 36

Spring Fling spring look, 142, _142_, **143**

Starbucks, 28

Stella McCartney Gentle Cleansing Milk, 50

Stevia, 32

Stila cosmetics, 12

Strawberries

    Berry Blast juice, 37

    Immune Zoom juice, 38

Stress and skin, 22

Sugar and skin, 31–33

Sukicolor

    Color Cream Lip/Cheek, _117_

    eye shadow, _79_

    liquid formula concealer, _71_

    mascara, _127_

    pure cream stain, _74_, _127_, _132_, _158_

    Rich Pigment mascara, _81_, _138_, _158_

Sula Nail Polish, 90

Summer makeup look, **144**, 145, _145_

Sunburn, 58–59, _110_

Sun exposure and aging, 56

Sun protection

    for men, 108, _108_, 110–11

    products, 57, _58_, 108, 110–11

    for women, 56–57, _57_

Sunscreen. _See also specific product_

    for body, _58_

    conventional, 57, 108

    eco-friendly, 110–11

    for face, _58_

    for men, 108, _108_, 110

    moisturizer with, 57

    skin allergies and, 57, 108

Sweet potatoes for healthy skin, 23

T

Tea bags for sunburn, 59

Teen makeup look, 147–48, **148**, _148_, **149**

Tetra Paks, 31

Thermos for water intake, 30

Thirties makeup look, 153–54, **154**, _154_, **155**

Tinted moisturizer, 67–68, _67_, 85

Tinting eyebrows, 83

Tomato juice for toning skin, _49_

Toning. _See also specific product_

    apple cider vinegar for, _53_

    chamomile for, _53_

    combination skin, 53, _53_

    dry skin, 51, _51_

    mint leaves for, _51_

    normal skin, 47, _47_

    oily skin, 49, _49_

    rose water for, _47_

    tomato juice for, _49_

    watermelon juice for, _49_

Toxins, 23, 30, 41

Trail mix, _22_

Turmeric, 34

Tweezers, _82_

Twenties makeup look, 147–48, **148**, _148_, **149**

U

USDA Organic logo, 6

V

Vanilla Chai Hand and Body Lotion, 55

Vegetables, _20_, 35. _See also specific type_

Vitamin A, 2, 23

Vitamin C, 2, 21–23, 32

Vitamin D, _57_

Vitamin E, 2, _9_, 21, _24_, 92

Vitamins, 2, 17. _See also specific type_

W

Walgreens, 13
Water intake
    on airplane, <u>27</u>
    coconut water and, 30–31
    diet and, 29–30
    energy and, 29–30
    plastic bottles of water and, 30
    skin and, 29–30
    thermos for, 30
Watermelon juice for toning skin, <u>49</u>
Water retention, <u>28</u>
Weight loss and sugar, 32
Weleda shaving cream, 100
Wide-set eyes, 79
Winter makeup look, **140**, 141, <u>141</u>
Wounds, skin, <u>55</u>

W (Wrinkles)

Wrinkles
    aging and, 20
    inevitability of, 20
    preventing
        cinnamon, 33
        oils, 24
        sweet potatoes, 23
    sugar and, 31
    sun exposure and, 56

Y

Yogurt
    for cleansing skin, <u>52</u>
    for exfoliation, <u>46</u>

Z

Zinc, 21
Zoya Nail Polish, 90